Magic Needles

Feel Younger And Live Longer With Acupuncture

Jun Xu , M.D., L.AC.
Frank Murray

16
EasyRead Large

RHYW

Copyright Page from the Original Book

The information contained in this book is based upon the research and personal and professional experiences of the authors. It is not intended as a substitute for consulting with your physician or other healthcare provider. Any attempt to diagnose and treat an illness should be done under the direction of a healthcare professional.

The publisher does not advocate the use of any particular healthcare protocol but believes the information in this book should be available to the public. The publisher and authors are not responsible for any adverse effects or consequences resulting from the use of the suggestions, preparations, or procedures discussed in this book. Should the reader have any questions concerning the appropriateness of any procedures or preparation mentioned, the authors and the publisher strongly suggest consulting a professional healthcare advisor.

Basic Health Publications, Inc.
28812 Top of the World Drive
Laguna Beach, CA 92651
949-715-7327 • www.basichealthpub.com

A Note about Authorship:
Chapters 1 and 2 are written by Frank Murray. Chapter 7 is jointly written by Frank Murray and Dr. Jun Xu. The remaining thirty-one chapters are written by Dr. Jun Xu.

Library of Congress Cataloging-in-Publication Data

Xu, Jun
Magic needles : feel younger and live longer with acupuncture / Jun Xu, and Frank Murray.
p. cm.
Includes bibliographical references and index.
ISBN 978-1-59120-222-6
1. Acupuncture. 2. Medicine, Chinese. I. Murray, Frank. II. Title.
RM184.X83 2011
615.8'92--dc23
2011018041

Editor: Roberta W. Waddell
Typesetting/Book design: Gary A. Rosenberg
Cover design: Mike Stromberg

Printed in the United States of America

10 9 8 7 6 5 4 3 2 1

TABLE OF CONTENTS

To our agent, Caroline Hutton, for her dedication and perseverance in getting this important book published

Acknowledgments

My grateful appreciation to the following people, who gave me encouragement and help. Without their support, it's unlikely this book would ever be presented to our readers. My thanks go to:

Norman Goldfind, my publisher, who gave me the opportunity to write a professional book for our general readers.

Roberta Waddell, my main editor, who spent months of days, nights, and weekends to make my professional language more readable to our lay audience, and who also gave me a lot of fascinating ideas about how to make the book better.

Melanie Chow, who helped me reshape my draft when she was an English student at Brown University.

Hong Su, L. Ac., my beloved wife, who is also a licensed acupuncturist—we trained together in Traditional Chinese Medicine in China. She read all my drafts, and gave me encouragement and many suggestions. Thanks to her endless efforts on my behalf, I finally finished this book, and for this, and everything else she does for me, I am indebted to her all my life.

Jun Xu, MD., L. Ac.

Foreword

Xin-Nons Li, MD, FACP

Integration of Chinese traditional medicine with Western practices is the goal of many physicians who are trained in China, and the author of this book, Dr. Jun Xu, is one such practitioner who has reached this goal.

I first met Dr. Jun Xu in 1996, more than fifteen years ago when we were both training as interns in Pittsburgh, PA. I was impressed that he had studied in two Chinese Traditional Medical Schools, Jiangxi College of Chinese Medicine, and Guangzhou College of Chinese Medicine, and had then done postgraduate study in Western medicine at both Albert Einstein College of Medicine in New York and the University of Georgia. In Pennsylvana, he continued his training as a resident in rehabilitation medicine while I pursued internal medicine. As a physician who was fully trained in both traditional Chinese medicine (TCM) and Western medicine, Dr. Xu was well prepared to integrate the two systems and he has done so since opening his clinic in 2000. This book is the summary of his practical experience these past ten years.

When I reviewed the manuscript, I found that *Magic Needles* is not only a highly useful source for people who seek alternative medicine, but is also a practical guide for medical practitioners. In Parts 1 and 2, Dr. Xu introduces, in layman's terms, a basic knowledge of Chinese traditional medicine and the details of acupuncture, which can help readers easily obtain a fundamental knowledge of TCM and acupuncture, including its history, theories, mechanisms, and current scientific evidence. By presenting this information in clear, simple language, general readers will understand why acupuncture works, which will give them the confidence to choose acupuncture as an effective alternate approach to their health.

In Part Tree, Dr. Xu illustrates his practical experience with acupuncture and Chinese traditional medicine to treat various medical conditions, from pain management to a common cold. Readers can quickly find chapters on different medical conditions and learn the TCM theories for these individual cases.

In last decade, more and more Americans have come to seek treatments from alternative methods. *Magic Needles* outlines a number of Dr. Xu's case histories from his ten years of practical experience integrating Chinese traditional medicine and Western medicine, and is a great source for those looking to be treated with Chinese traditional medicine and acupuncture, as well as for those practicing acupuncture in the Western world.

Xin-Nong Li, MD, FACP
Associate Clinical Professor of Medicine
School of Medicine, University of California, Davis

Foreword

Marc Brodsky, MD, MBA, MPH

How may YOU optimize your quality of life and enhance your sense of well-being? For answers to this question, Dr. Xu's *Magic Needles* is a must read.

During my tour as a Navy Physician in Japan, my patients who visited Eastern Medicine practitioners in the community introduced me to a tradition of medicine very different from my conventional medical training. I first observed acupuncture being done on one of my patients who had injured his back in a motor scooter accident. The effect of the first treatment was dramatic, and although the patient ultimately underwent surgery, he was able to get substantial relief from his suffering through the combination of medications, physical therapy, and repeated sessions with the tiny needles that were placed in his lower back and attached to electrical current.

The synergism of different systems of medicine became more apparent as I learned more about the philosophy and treatments of Eastern Medicine. Transformed by my exposure to Eastern Medicine, I completed a fellowship in East-West Medicine at the University of California Los Angeles (UCLA) and went on to pursue this ancient (to me, innovative) model of healthcare.

Like some of my mentors at UCLA, Dr. Xu earned a Medical Doctor degree in both Chinese medicine and conventional medicine. In this book, Dr. Xu draws from his expertise in multiple medical disciplines to explain the diagnosis and treatment of common health conditions from both conventional medicine and Chinese medicine perspectives.

The easy-to-read history and overview of Chinese medicine will assist even those readers with no experience in Chinese medicine. Each recommended acupuncture point is clearly identified on the photographic image of a live model. Lifestyle self-care strategies are also a part of the care plan of each condition. Engaging stories of actual patients exemplify how Chinese medicine and conventional medicine may work together to solve challenging problems in a holistic way that is safe and scientifically informed.

So, delay no longer and start reading now. Dr. Xu's *Magic Needles,* along with standard medical care and self-care will empower you to be your own *number one* advocate for health and wellness.

Marc Brodsky, MD, MBA, MPH
Assistant Professor of Clinical Medicine, Columbia University, New York, NY
Medical Director, Center for Integrative Medicine and Wellness at Stamford Hospital, Stamford, CT

PART ONE

The Importance of Acupuncture

Acupuncture releases a natural energy that can alleviate even long-standing health conditions. Pain-free acupuncture is, therefore, an ideal treatment for asthma, bronchitis, depression, drug and alcohol addiction headaches, smoking, women's health problems, and much more.

Since acupuncture is not a self-help treatment as such (where as acupressure can be), but requires a practitioner you may want to take this book with you to show the acupuncturist the chapter that corresponds to your condition. Included is valuable information on the techniques involved, and in the Appendix, there is a chapter-by-chapter list of tips to acupuncturists for each of the twenty-three conditions covered in this thorough book.

1

In the Beginning

In traditional Chinese medicine (TCM), acupuncture and moxibustion are important procedures that prevent and treat disease, either by puncturing certain points on the body with needles, or by applying heat with ignited moxa wool, reported *Essentials of Chinese Acupuncture,* a translation of *Zhongguo Zhenjiuxue Gaiyao.* Requiring simple equipment, they have been widely popular in China and elsewhere for thousands of years.[1]

"The initiation and development of the art of acupuncture and moxibustion have a long historical process," the publication said. "They are summaries of experience of the Chinese laboring people of many centuries in their struggle against disease. As early as the Stone Age, people used needles fashioned of stone for curative purposes. These are known as *Bian Shi* and are a rudiment of acupuncture."

When humans entered the Bronze and then the Iron Age, needles made of these metals were substituted for the stone Bian Shi. With the development of more advanced techniques, needling instruments were constantly improved, providing further refinement of acupuncture.

Moxibustion originated after man's introduction of fire. It is assumed that, while warming themselves by the fire, people in ancient times accidentally found relief or disappearance of certain pain or illness when definite areas of the skin were subjected to burning. Moxa leaves *(Artemisia vulgaris* or mugwort) were later chosen as the material for cauterization since they are easily lit, and the heat is mild and effective in removing obstruction in channels and collaterals.

The earliest medical classic in China, *Huangdi Neijing (Canon of Medicine)* was compiled between 500–300B.C., the publication added. It is a summary of the medical experience and theoretical knowledge prior to the Warring States period (475–221B.C.). The book, which consists of two parts —*Suwen* and *Ling-shu*— describes the basic theories of traditional Chinese medicine, such as yin-yang, the five elements, zang-fu, channels and collaterals, qi (vital energy) and blood, etiology, pathology, diagnostic methods, and differentiation of syndromes, as well as basic knowledge concerning acupuncture points and needling methods.

The Warring States period in China, and later in Japan, was a period in which small feuding kingdoms, or fiefdoms, struggled for supremacy. The Chinese Warring States period was dominated by six or seven small feuding Chinese kingdoms. It was the age of Confucian thinkers, Mencius and Zunzi.[2]

Following *Neijing,* there appeared quite a number of treatises on acupuncture and moxibustion written in different dynasties, with representative ones being:[1]

Zhenjiu Jiayijing (A Classic of Acupuncture and Moxibustion, 265A.D.), compiled by Huangfu Mi of the Jin Dynasty.

Tongren Shuxue Zhenjiu Tujing (Illustrated Manual on Points for Acupuncture and Moxibustion Shown on a Bronze Figure, 1026A.D.), compiled by Wang Weiyi, an acupuncturist of the Song Dynasty. The next year, Wang Weiyi sponsored the casting of two life-size bronze figures marked with acupuncture points, a momentous event in the development of acupuncture and moxibustion.

Zhenjiu Zishengjing (A Classic of Acupuncture and Moxibustion Therapy, 1220A.D.), compiled by Wang Zhizhong of the Song Dynasty.

Shisijing Fahui (The Enlargement of the Fourteen Channels, 1341A.D.), a work by Hua Boren of the Yuan Dynasty).

Zhenjiu Dacheng (Compendium of Acupuncture and Moxibustion, 1601A.D.), a work by Yang Jizhou, an acupuncturist of the Ming Dynasty. It has been an indispensable reference book in studying acupuncture and moxibustion in the almost four centuries since it was published.

Chinese acupuncture and moxibustion were introduced to Korea and Japan in the Sixth Century when a monk named Zhi Cong traveled Eastward by sea carrying copies of *Mingtangtu (Illustrated Manual of Channels, Collaterals and Acupuncture Points), Zhenjiu Jiayijing,* and other medical books.

In the late Seventeenth Century, acupuncture and moxibustion spread to Europe. This actively promoted the medical and cultural exchange between China and other countries in the world. As reported elsewhere in this book, acupuncture is rapidly gaining popularity in the United States.

2

The Increasing Popularity of Acupuncture

Interest in acupuncture in the United States took a big step forward in 1971, when Henry Kissinger, Secretary of State under President Richard M. Nixon, visited China. Kissinger was accompanied by James Reston, a reporter for *The New York Times,* who had an attack of appendicitis that Chinese doctors treated surgically, using acupuncture as an anesthesia. Reston's subsequent article in *The Times* generated considerable interest in acupuncture.[1]

The use of acupuncture has become more and more popular and mainstream because the therapy taps into the body's own *pharmacy* and helps the body's ability to heal itself. While Western medicine deals with treating individuals in parts, acupuncture addresses how illnesses are related to one another.[2]

The therapy has been shown to affect specific areas of the brain associated with stress, drug addiction, and chronic pain, and it can assist in the side effects of cancer treatment. Acupuncture can diminish pain and inflammation and provide a preventive benefit by keeping inflammation from recurring. There is clear evidence for the benefits of acupuncture in treating a variety of conditions, including alcohol and drug addiction, anxiety, carpal tunnel syndrome, constipation, diarrhea, gastritis, headaches, insomnia, and lower back pain. In addition, research has shown how acupuncture may be beneficial in treating attention deficit hyperactivity disorder (ADHD), mild anxiety, and osteoarthritis.

Approximately one-half of those with headaches respond to acupuncture, as do about one-third of those with trigeminal neuralgia (trigeminal relates to the fifth cranial nerve). It can also relieve those with post-stroke spasticity.

Other conditions where the use of acupuncture can be beneficial include nausea, and even Raynaud's Phenomenon. In these, and all conditions, there is a low incidence of adverse effects using acupuncture when compared to medical procedures or therapeutic drugs.

In the past three decades, acupuncture has begun to be integrated into Western medical applications. Relief from pain without anesthetics is the best known and most frequently used application of acupuncture.[3]

There are different types of acupuncture, including traditional Chinese acupuncture, auricular acupuncture, French energetics acupuncture, and Korean and Japanese acupuncture. In the U.S., requirements for administering acupuncture vary from state to state, from 100 hours of specialized training to a four-year program.

Much of what were once perceived as alternative therapies are now regarded by mainstream medicine as adjuncts to traditional Western medicine. For example, patient-oriented care is the new emphasis that seeks to enhance the patient's own attitudes and emotional resources to promote healing. The reason for the spark in interest for such modalities as acupuncture is that many who are ill have needs that go beyond current medicine's technology.[4]

Increased information and awareness of older medical systems, such as TCM and acupuncture, offers benefits to many people. There is the perception that contemporary Western medicine has reduced healing to a mechanical process, and has failed to acknowledge the spiritual and psychological component of life.

Doctors who practice it often use acupuncture as another therapeutic modality of general medicine.[5]

The American Academy of Medical Acupuncture, established in 1987 in Los Angeles, California, requires its members to have at least 200 hours of training in a continuing medical-education approved program. While the academy is open to all physicians, most of them are interested in pain management. Anesthesiologists and orthopedic surgeons have also taken the course to control pain.[6]

How does acupuncture work? Some studies suggest a release of endorphins as one possibility. These are a group of proteins with potent analgesic properties. Another immune response suggests that inserting needles may alter the balance between the sympathetic and parasympathetic nervous systems.

Glen S. Rothfield, an M.D. from Arlington, Massachusetts, uses acupuncture and natural medicine in his practice. As an example, Rothfield treats arthritis with niacinimide (vitamin B3), bioflavonoids, willow bark, and acupuncture before he resorts to nonsteroidal and anti-inflammatory drugs.[1]

Andrew Weil, M.D., a Tucson, Arizona physician, said that people who come to him seeking alternative care are highly intelligent, motivated, and educated. He practices natural and preventive medicine, which includes nutritional medicine, diet therapy, vitamins and minerals, and mind-body approaches. He reports that 10 percent of his patients are well and see him only for preventive and lifestyle counseling. About forty-five percent come to him for routine conditions, such as allergies, anxiety, digestive disorders, headaches, insomnia, and sinus infections, and acupuncture is one of the methods he uses to ameliorate these conditions.

One main reason for the increasing popularity of alternative medicine, including acupuncture, is that it is being sought out by physicians who are frustrated with the system they are being taught, and there is a huge patient interest in it. For at least one-fourth of the world's population, acupuncture is more commonly used than aspirin.

Alternative therapies can reduce costs in a number of ways, since many hospitalizations are due to harmful drug interactions resulting from conventionally prescribed drugs.

Some people prefer visits to physicians because they are looking for emotional support and guidance, not necessarily treatment for a specific illness. But alternative therapies, including acupuncture, can provide that kind of support at a much lower cost, and they also stress prevention.

3

How Acupuncture Works

ACUPUNCTURE FROM THE PERSPECTIVE OF TRADITIONAL CHINESE MEDICINE

Acupuncture is one of the most important therapeutic tools in traditional Chinese medicine (TCM). According to TCM, there is a system of balance between our universal and human bodies, called yin and yang balance, with yin representing the feminine, night, winter, weak, dark, for example, and yang representing the masculine, day, summer, strong, light, and so on. Our bodies adjust this balance according to the changes in nature—for instance, when the sun rises in the morning, the yang in the body increases in order to provide the essential energy needed to perform daily activities, and when evening comes, the body's yin increases to accomodate that time of day.

There are fourteen major meridians within the body. Qi, the vital energy, circulates through these fourteen major meridians and numerous other tiny meridians in the body. Approximately 400 acupuncture points are found along these meridians. If there is an imbalance of yin and yang, the qi will be blocked along the meridian, and an illness will likely arise.

Fortunately, the ancient Chinese invented TCM to counteract this imbalance. The therapeutic tools of TCM include acupuncture, herbs, massage, moxa (a method for burning moxa to transfer energy from the burning herb to human body), qi gong (an energy/breathing exercise), and many others. Acupuncture needles can be inserted into any of the 400 specific points in the body to open the blockage and help the body balance its yin and yang, thereby treating and healing the illness.

A report from the Consensus Development Conference on Acupuncture held at the National Institutes of Health (N.I.H.) in 1997 stated that acupuncture is "widely practiced [...] by thousands of physicians, dentists, acupuncturists, and other practitioners—for relief or prevention of pain and for various other health conditions."[1]

According to the 2007 National Health Interview Survey (NHIS), which included a comprehensive survey of complementary and alternative medicine use by Americans, "an estimated 3.1 million adults and 150,000 Children had used acupuncture in the previous year. Between the 2002 and 2007 NHIS's, acupuncture use among adults had increased by three-tenths of 1 percent (approximately one million people)."[2]

ACUPUNCTURE FROM THE PERSPECTIVES OF SCIENTIFIC THEORIES AND MECHANISMS OF ACTION

Two current major theories explain the mechanisms of acupuncture—the gate-control theory of pain and the neurohormonal theory.

Gate-Control Theory of Pain

In 1962, Ronald Melzack and P.D. Wall proposed the gate-control theory, which suggested that pain perception is not simply a direct response to the stimulation of pain fibers, but is also mediated by the cooperation of excitation and inhibition in pain pathways. Because the pain is controlled by the inhibitory action on the pain pathway, the *perception of pain can be altered.* In other words, *the pain can be gated on or off through various methods—mechanically, pharmacologically, physically, physiologically, and psychologically.*[3][4]

In 1976, Melzack used the gate-control theory to explain the mechanisms of acupuncture. He believed that acupuncture acts on the reticular formation in the brain stem to alter the pain pathway.[5]

This loosely organized area of the brain is involved in the waking and sleeping cycle and appears to be at the crux of basic neurological and behavioral functions of the human being.

Since Melzack's proposal, the gate-control theory has become more popular, and many studies have supported this theory about the mechanisms of acupuncture. Melzack's idea led to the theory of central control of pain gating, which proposes that pain is blockaded at the brain (i.e. central to the brain rather than at the spinal cord or periphery) via the release of endogenous opioids (natural painkillers in the brain), and neurohormones, such as endorphins and enkephalins (naturally occurring morphines).[6][7][8]

Neurohormonal Theory, a Contemporary Acupuncture Model

Based on information from the gate-control theory, many scientists began to study the central neurotransmitters, such as endorphins (i.e. opioids and nitric oxide, an important messenger molecule involved in many physiological and pathological processes that can be both beneficial and detrimental), and their regulation in many other levels of the brain along the pain pathways, including the periaqueductal gray (an area of the brain involved in the regulation of pain), the thalamus (a centrally-located structure that controls the flow of all information to the cortex), and the feedback pathways from the cerebral cortex to the thalamus. Pain blockade at these brain locations is often mediated by neurohormones, especially those that bind to the opioid receptors (the pain-blockade site).[9][10]

Recently, scientists have started to use fMRI (functional magnetic resonance imaging) and PET (positron emission tomography) to study the mechanism of acupuncture. These studies have shown that the pain reduction by acupuncture may be mediated through decreased activities of several parts of the brain—the thalamus, the insula, and the anterior cingulate cortex.[11][12][13] The insula is a receiving zone that reads the physiological state of the entire body and then generates subjective feelings that can bring about actions, like eating, that keep the body in a state of internal balance. Information from the insula is relayed to other brain structures that appear to be involved in decision-making, especially the anterior cingulate and prefrontal cortices.

4

Illnesses that Acupuncture Can Treat

ACUPUNCTURE FROM THE TRADITIONAL CHINESE MEDICINE PERSPECTIVE

In ancient China, with no Western medicine, the Chinese were able to endure serious weather and environmental conditions with the help of such traditional Chinese medicine as acupuncture that protected and improved their health and well-being.

According to TCM, the body's internal organs and meridians control all human activities. Clinically, pathological phenomena are reflections of the pathology of the internal organs and meridians. By identifying the diseases that belong to any internal organs or meridians, acupuncturists can select the correct meridians, internal organs, and acupuncture points. The disease can then be treated, and most likely cured, through acupuncture.

The following diseases or illnesses have been treated with acupuncture for thousands of years.

Internal Medicine Illnesses

- Abdominal ache
- Chronic cough or acute cough
- Abdominal hernia
- Diarrhea
- Asthma
- Common cold
- Constipation
- Edema (swelling)
- Heart palpitations
- Impotence
- Insomnia
- Jaundice
- Lung disease
- Malaria
- Nocturnal emissions
- Rectal prolapse (condition where rectum falls outside the body)
- Stomach ache
- Vomiting

OB/GYN and Childhood Illnesses

- ADHD (attention deficit and hyperactive disease)
- Amenorrhea (absence of a menstrual period for at least three consecutive months)
- Cerebral palsy
- Dysmenorrhea (severe uterine pain during menstruation)

- Fetal breech (fetus lies with the buttocks or feet closest to the cervix instead of the head)
- Fetal stasis (a slowing or stoppage of the normal flow of a bodily fluid)
- Lack of milk
- Postpolio
- Unreasonable infertility
- Urinary incontinence
- Uterine bleeding, including metrorrhagia (uterine bleeding at irregular intervals, particularly between expected menstrual periods), and metrostaxis (slight but continuous uterine hemorrhage)

Ear, Nose, and Throat Diseases

- Eye pain
- Nearsightedness
- Sinusiti
- Sore throat
- Tinnitus and deafness
- Toothache

Bone and Joint, Muscle, and Nerve Diseases

Bone and Joint

- All osteoarthritis at neck, shoulder, elbow, wrist, lower back, hip, knee, and ankle.

Muscle

Ankle and foot

- Sprain and Achilles tendon sprain and tendonitis, plantar fasciitis, Morton's neuroma

Elbow

- Bursitis, tendonitis
- Triceps tendonitis, sprain

Hip

- Bursitis, hamstring strain, and tendonitis
- Bursitis hip strain, groin strain

Knee

- Biker's knee, jumper's knee, runner's knee, and shin splints
- Meniscus injuries and sprain

Shoulder

- Frozen shoulder
- Tears
- Joint sprain
- Joint injury
- Rotator cuff tear, and rotator cuff tendonitis
- Tendonitis and rupture of biceps

Wrist and Hand

- Dupuytren's contracture (condition causing tightening of connective tissue in the hand; fingers can become permanently bent down and function of hand is impaired)
- Trigger finger, Jersey finger, mallet finger

Nerves

- Carpal tunnel syndrome
- Cervical and lumbar sacral radiculopathy (compressed nerve in the spine that can cause pain, numbness, tingling, or weakness along the course of the nerve)
- Dizziness
- Facial paralysis
- Headaches
- Hypertension
- Parkinson's disease
- Strokes
- Trigeminal neuralgia (chronic pain condition that affects the trigeminal nerve in the face and is characterized by episodes of extreme, sporadic, sudden burning or shock-like face pain)
- Rheumatic Diseases
- Ankylosing spondylitis (long-term disease causing joint inflammation between spinal bones, and between spine and pelvis, eventually resulting in affected spinal bones joining together)
- Crohn's disease and ulcerative colitis-induced arthritis
- Gout
- Juvenile rheumatoid arthritis
- Mixed connective tissue disorder
- Psoriatic arthritis (autoimmune disease in which a person has both psoriasis and arthritis; psoriasis generally manifests as patches of raised red skin with scales, and arthritis is joint inflammation)

- Rheumatoid arthritis

5

Acupuncture Treatments Approved or Recommended by Physicians, the W.H.O., and the N.I.H.

PHYSICIANS

In 1987, the American Academy of Medical Acupuncture (A.A.M.A.) was founded by a group of physicians who graduated from the Medical Acupuncture for Physicians training program sponsored by the School of Medicine at UCLA. The A.A.M.A. is the sole physician-only, professional acupuncture society in North America. Its members come from diverse training backgrounds and represent all the disciplines of medical acupuncture currently practiced in the United States and Canada.

Many patients often ask their doctors if acupuncture can realistically improve an illness or medical condition. The A.A.M.A. suggests that acupuncture can be an effective treatment if administered by an experienced practitioner. For example, doctors should look closely at their patient's medical history, condition, and past treatments in order to conclude whether acupuncture can be a suitable treatment by itself or as an adjunctive therapy.

A physician from the A.A.M.A. said, "I generally tell patients that if their treatment, according to a Western diagnosis with options, is not resolving the problem, is quite expensive, or has significant side effects/hassles associated with it, then clearly acupuncture is worth a try. I include the Western diagnosis criteria because I think, as just an example, it is ridiculous to treat someone's dizziness with acupuncture if what they need is to have excessive wax cleaned out from their ear canals. On the other hand, if one is having difficulty controlling or improving asthma with Western treatments, a trial of acupuncture makes utmost sense."[1]

THE W.H.O.

These are the conditions recommended for acupuncture by the World Health Organization (W.H.O.).[1]

Bronchopulmonary Diseases

- Acute bronchitis
- Bronchial asthma

Disorders of the Mouth Cavity

- Gingivitis
- Pain after tooth extraction
- Pharyngitis

- Toothache

Eye Disorders

- Acute conjuctivitis
- Cataracts (without complications)
- Central retinitis
- Myopia

Gastrointestinal Disorders

- Acute and chronic colitis
- Acute and chronic gastritis
- Acute bacterial dysentery
- Chronic duodenal ulcer
- Constipation
- Diarrhea
- Gastric hyperacidity
- Gastroptosis (abnormal downward displacement of stomach frequently causing digestive symptoms and constipation)
- Hiccups
- Spasm of the esophagus

Neurological Disorders

- Facial paralysis
- Headaches
- Intercostal neuralgia
- Ménière's syndrome (disorder of the inner ear affecting hearing and balance)
- Migraine

- Neurogenic bladder dysfunction (malfunctioning bladder due to interference with nerves associated with urination)
- Nocturnal enuresis (bedwetting)
- Paralysis after apoplectic fit
- Paralysis caused by poliomyelitis
- Peripheral neuropathy
- Trigeminal neuralgia

Orthopedic Disorders

- Low back pain
- Rheumatoid arthritis
- Sciatica
- Tennis elbow

Respiratory Diseases

- Acute rhinitis
- Acute sinusitis
- Acute tonsillitis
- Common cold

THE N.I.H

The National Institutes of Health (N.I.H.) held its first meeting on acupuncture from November 3–5, 1997, with twelve members forming an acupuncture panel. After the meeting, they issued the following statement expressing the N.I.H. views on acupuncture.

"Acupuncture as a therapeutic intervention is widely practiced in the United States. While there have been many studies of its potential usefulness, many of these studies provide equivocal results because of design, sample size, and other factors. The issue is further complicated by inherent difficulties in the use of appropriate controls, such as placebos and sham acupuncture groups. However, promising results have emerged, for example, showing efficacy of acupuncture in adult postoperative and chemotherapy nausea and vomiting and in postoperative dental pain. There are other situations, such as addiction, asthma, carpal tunnel syndrome, fibromyalgia, headaches, low back pain, menstrual cramps, myofascial pain, osteoarthritis, stroke rehabilitation, and tennis elbow, in which acupuncture may be useful as an adjunct treatment, or an acceptable alternative, or be included in a comprehensive management program. Further research is likely to uncover additional areas where acupuncture interventions will be useful."[2]

6

Acupuncture Research

RECENT PROGRESS IN RESEARCHING CONDITIONS SUITABLE FOR ACUPUNCTURE TREATMENT

Because the N.I.H. has not held a meeting since 1997 to discuss new medical research and knowledge that has accumulated over the past thirteen years, this chapter will review recent published findings about the effectiveness of acupuncture and the various illnesses it can treat.

Acupuncture Treatment for Carpal Tunnel Syndrome (CTS)

- Two methods were used to treat seventy-seven people affected by mild-to-moderate carpal tunnel syndrome. The first method was more mainstream and included steroids: two weeks of prednisolone, 20mg daily, followed by two weeks of prednisolone, 10mg daily. The second method employed traditional Chinese medicine: acupuncture administered in eight sessions over four weeks. A questionnaire was used as a subjective measurement to rate the five major symptoms (pain, numbness, paresthesia, weakness/clumsiness, and nocturnal awakening) on a scale from 0 (no symptoms) to 10 (very severe). The total score of the five categories was termed the global symptom score (GSS). At weeks two and four of treatment, both groups experienced an improvement in their GSS. Furthermore, the acupuncture group showed a significant decrease in nocturnal awakening and a decrease in distal motor latency at week four. The results suggest that short-term acupuncture treatment is as effective as short-term low-dose prednisolone for mild-to-moderate CTS and can be an effective alternative choice.[1]

Acupuncture Treatment for Hip or Knee Pain

- A study of 3,633 people with chronic osteoarthritis-associated hip or knee pain illustrated that acupuncture treatments led to pronounced quality-of-life improvements. Based on the Western Ontario and McMaster Universities Osteoarthritis Index (WOMAC) pain and function scores, the improvement was evident as early as three months after treatment and lasted for at least six months. Thus, the study suggests that acupuncture plus routine care can lead to a significant clinical improvement.[2]
- Two groups of 570 people with osteoarthritis of the knee were studied. The control group received

either six two-hour sham acupuncture sessions over twelve weeks, or twenty-three sham acupuncture sessions over twenty-six weeks. Those receiving true acupuncture received twenty-three sessions over twenty-six weeks. Overall, the participants in the true acupuncture group had higher improvement in the Western Ontario and McMaster Universities Osteoarthritis Index (WOM-AC) pain and function scores. This suggests that acupuncture can provide improvement in function and pain relief as an adjunctive therapy for osteoarthritis of the knee.[3]

Acupuncture Treatment for Impotence

The ancient Chinese found that acupuncture was also an effective treatment for impotence, and recent medical studies have proven this true.

- Twenty-nine men with purely psychogenic impotence were treated with a varying number of acupuncture sessions. Following the acupuncture treatments, twenty of the twenty-nine men demonstrated successful erections, suggesting that acupuncture may be an effective alternative for managing impotence.[4]
- In another study, twenty-two men with psychogenic erectile dysfunction (pED) were randomized into two treatment groups: acupuncture specific against ED (treatment group) or acupuncture

specific against headaches (placebo group). In the treatment group, 68.4 percent of the subjects had a satisfactory response and another 21.05 percent had improved erections (measured through treatment with 50gm of sildenafil). Overall, the study suggests that acupuncture can be an effective treatment for those with pED.[5]

Acupuncture Treatment for Infertility

For women

Many studies have recently revealed that acupuncture may greatly improve the success rate of in-vitro fertilization.

- At a university in-vitro fertilization (IVF) center in Germany, 225 infertile women undergoing IVF or Intra Cytoplasmic Sperm Injection (ICSI) were separated into two treatment groups and given luteal-phase acupuncture according to the principles of traditional Chinese medicine, or placebo acupuncture. Those who received the luteal-phase acupuncture had significantly higher clinical pregnancy and ongoing pregnancy rates (33.6 percent and 28.4 percent, respectively) than the placebo group (15.6 percent and 13.8 percent), thereby suggesting that acupuncture has a positive effect on the outcome of IVF/ICSI.[6]
- A later study on 1,366 women undergoing IVF confirmed the above results. If the embryo-

transfer process was complemented with acupuncture, the rate of clinical pregnancy and subsequent number of live births was significantly increased.[7]

- Another study of sixty-seven women undergoing IVF sheds light on the biological reasons for acupunctures effectiveness. Blood samples were taken from the women in order to measure their serum corticosterone (CORT) and serum prolactin (PRL) levels. The group that received acupuncture had significantly higher levels of CORT and PRL compared with the control group, suggesting that acupuncture increases the trend toward more normal fertile cycle dynamics.[8]

For men

Acupuncture can also treat infertility that arises due to a low sperm count.

- Twenty-eight infertile men with severe oligoasthenozoospermia received TCM acupuncture and twenty-nine infertile men received placebo acupuncture. A higher percentage of motile sperm (but no effect on sperm concentration), was found after acupuncture, compared with placebo acupuncture.[9]
- Another study illustrated that acupuncture treatments can increase sperm count. Infertile men who received acupuncture were found to have a decreased scrotal skin temperature and an increased sperm count.[10]

Acupuncture for Low Back Pain

- Over a period of seven weeks, 638 adults with chronic mechanical low back pain were given ten treatments of either individualized acupuncture, standardized acupuncture, stimulated acupuncture, or usual care (i.e. pain medication, rest, application of heating pads, etc). After seven weeks, the individualized, standardized, and stimulated acupuncture groups reported significant improvements compared with the usual care group (symptoms improved by 1.6 to 1.9 points in the treatment groups compared with 0.7 points in the usual care group). Similar results were found after one year.[11]

Acupuncture Treatment for Nausea and Vomiting after Chemotherapy and/or an Operation

Many patients undergoing chemotherapy and/or an operation experience nausea and vomiting. Unfortunately, few effective treatments exist for these symptoms. Throughout history, acupuncture has been shown to decrease nausea and vomiting very effectively. Recent studies have been done on the effectiveness of acupuncture for these symptoms that arise post-chemotherapy and post-operation.

- **Post-chemotherapy.** Eleven trials of 1,247 men and women were pooled together to study the effectiveness of acupuncture-point stimulation (electroacupuncture) on acute and delayed chemotherapy-induced nausea and vomiting in those with cancer. Although further studies need to be done to conclude the clinical relevance of acupuncture in comparison to current pharmacologic antiemetic therapies, researchers found that acupuncture-point stimulation reduced acute vomiting, and that self-administered acupressure also led to a protective effect for acute nausea.[12]

- **Post-operative nausea and vomiting (PONV).** In twenty-six trials of 3,347 post-operative patients, it was demonstrated that stimulation of the acupuncture point P6, manually or with electricity, led to significant reductions in nausea and vomiting post-operatively if the patients are not administered antiemetic prophylaxis drugs (used to prevent or alleviate nausea and vomiting). If these drugs are administered, the P6 acupoint stimulation still helps reduce the risk of nausea, but not the vomiting.[13]

Acupuncture for Neck Pain

- In a study published in May 2009, nearly fifty people received either active or sham electrical acustimulation of the wrist at specified acupuncture points, and also completed a thirty-minute routine of standardized neck exercises. The acustimulation was administered for thirty minutes, twice a week for four weeks. Those in the study reported a significant reduction in chronic neck pain, and the effects lasted at least one month post-treatment.[14]

- After reviewing all acupuncture studies published in China and the rest of the world since February 2006, Trinh et al. found ten trials that examined acupuncture treatments for chronic neck pain. Overall, the studies illustrated that acupuncture relieves pain better than some sham treatments, and people who received acupuncture reported less pain during their short-term follow-ups. It is also evident that acupuncture is more effective than inactive treatments for relieving pain post-treatment.[15]
- One hundred seventy-seven people between eighteen and eighty-five-years-old who were experiencing chronic neck pain were randomly allocated five treatments over three weeks with acupuncture, massage, or sham laser acupuncture. The study concluded that acupuncture was the most effective treatment for chronic neck pain and that the positive results were not due to a placebo effect.[16]

Acupuncture Treatment for Rheumatoid Arthritis

Further research is needed to produce definite and consistent results on the effectiveness of acupuncture in treating rheumatoid arthritis, but current clinical studies have already demonstrated acupuncture's therapeutic potential.

- A functional evaluation study after acupuncture treatment suggests that acupuncture relieves symptoms, remedies physical functions, and can improve the quality of life in people with rheumatoid arthritis (acupuncture has little to no anti-inflammatory benefits). Overall, the study by Sato et al. shows that acupuncture can be used for therapeutic mechanisms.[17]

  Chinese physicians conducted a study on 100 people with rheumatoid arthritis, splitting them into a standard medication group and a bee-venom group. Those in the control group were given Methotrexate, Sulfasalazine, and Meloxicam. The bee-venom group was treated with 1) bee-stings at the *Ashi* points, and 2) the above-mentioned Western medicines. The study showed the combined application of the bee-venom therapy *and* mainstream medicine to be more effective for rheumatoid arthritis than simply using Western drugs. In addition, with the use of bee-venom therapy, the dosage of the Western medicines can be reduced and the overall relapse rate is lower.[18]

Acupuncture for Shoulder Pain

- In twelve treatments administered over a six-week period, thirty-one adults diagnosed with osteoarthritis, who had experienced chronic shoulder pain for at least eight weeks, were given three forms of treatment: individualized acupuncture points according to the approaches of traditional Chinese medicine; fixed, standard acupuncture points conventionally used for shoulder pain; and sham non-penetrating acupuncture. Overall, the study found clinically significant improvements in the acupuncture groups, with no difference between the individualized vs. the standardized treatment.[19]

Acupuncture Treatment for Smoking Cessation

Smoking and drug addiction are very important topics and many studies have been done in relation to acupuncture therapy.

- A study of 141 adult smokers used various combinations of three treatments: acupuncture, sham acupuncture, and education. Although all groups showed significant reductions in smoking and cigarette consumption, the combined acupuncture-education group was affected the most positively.[20]

Acupuncture Treatment for Strokes

- Within ten days of having a stroke, sixty-two post-stroke people were divided into three treatment groups: transcutaneous electrical stimulation (acupuncture), placebo stimulation, or standard rehabilitation alone. The stimulation was applied to four acupuncture points in the affected lower leg for one hour, five days a week for three weeks. Compared with standard rehabilitation and placebo stimulation, the transcutaneous electrical stimulation (TENS) to specified acupuncture points was the most effective treatment: this group had increased normal tone and more strength in the upward movement of the foot at the ankle, and decreased muscle spasms in the paralyzed limbs. These people also began walking two to four days earlier.[21]

Acupuncture Treatment for Tennis Elbow

- After reviewing ten years of online data of acupuncture treatment for lateral epicondylitis (tennis elbow), Trinh et al. determined that six studies were of a high quality (according to the Jadad scale) and that the data could be synthesized into an overall conclusion. The research suggested that acupuncture is an effective treatment for the short-term relief of tennis elbow.[22]

7

How to Select an Acupuncturist

An acupuncture session usually involves a series of weekly or biweekly treatments in an outpatient setting, explained Mayo Clinic Health Information, Rochester, Minnesota. However, it is to have up to twelve treatments in total. While each practitioner has his or her own unique style, each visit usually involves an examination and an assessment of your health problem, the insertion of needles, and a discussion of self-care tips. A typical visit usually requires keeping the needles in the person's body about fifteen to thirty minutes. You should allocate around forty-five minutes to one hour per visit to finish all the procedures.[1]

Before the needles are inserted, you will lie in a comfortable position. Depending on where the needles are placed, you will lie face down, face up, or on your side. And depending on the experience of the acupuncturist, who always treats with single-use, sterile needles, you may occasionally feel a brief, sharp sensation when the needle is inserted, but generally the procedure is painless. If the practitioner is skillful in inserting the needles quickly through the skin, you will not usually feel pain when the needles penetrate the skin. It is, however, sometimes common to feel a deep, aching sensation when the needle reaches the intended depth.

After placement, the needles are sometimes gently moved or stimulated with electricity or heat, which is referred to as moxa, a burning Chinese herb around the handle of the needles. As many as thirty or more needles may need to be placed for each treatment. Once the needles are inserted, they are usually left in place for fifteen to thirty minutes.

Acupuncture is safe when performed properly, it has few side effects, and it is often used to complement other treatment options. It helps to control certain types of pain, and it may be a good alternative if you don't respond to pain medications or do not wish to take them.

If you are considering acupuncture, do the same things you would in choosing a doctor.

- Ask people you trust for recommendations.
- Check the practitioner's training and credentials.

THE FOUR TYPES OF ACUPUNCTURISTS PRACTICING IN THE UNITED STATES

Two Groups of Acupuncturists are M.D.'s

1. One group is licensed M.D. physicians with regular acupuncture training from China. There are many U.S.-licensed M.D. physicians graduated from Chinese medical schools who are currently practicing in the states. They have usually undergone five years of education, including both Western medicine and Chinese medicine in China. The students usually go for clinic internship and resident training in both a Western hospital and one for Chinese medicine. The medical school graduates are qualified to take the United States Medical License Examination after they finish at least three years residency training in the U.S., and they are then licensed to practice medicine in the U.S. Many of them have sound foundations for acupuncture practice. In many states, it is not necessary for M.D. physicians to have an acupuncture license to practice acupuncture.
2. A second group is acupuncturists practicing in the United States who are licensed M.D. physicians with regular acupuncture training from the United States. The UCLA School of Medicine offers a 300-

hour acupuncture course for M.D. physicians, which has been taught regularly since 1983. Six thousand physicians have completed this comprehensive program, and it has earned the reputation of conscientiously accomplishing its goal of creating clinically competent physician acupuncturists who can integrate acupuncture with conventional medicine. For more information, visit their website at: www.cme.ucla.edu/courses

There are many other programs accredited by the American Academy of Medical Acupuncture (A.A.M.A.) that offer similar programs to M.D. physicians. Their website: www.medicalacupuncture.org/aama_marf/aama.html lists A.A.M.A. board-certified physician acupuncturists in your state.

Two Groups are Non-Physician Acupuncturists

Most states require that non-physician acupuncturists pass an examination conducted by the National Certification Commission for Acupuncture and Oriental Medicine (NCCAOM): www.nccaom.org/

1. One group of non-physician practititioners is acupuncturists trained in the United States. These students must have their bachelor degrees before getting into the acupuncture schools in the U.S. They need at least three years of study for acupuncture, including a basic knowledge of TCM acupuncture, and a clinical rotation. After three

years of study, the graduates are qualified to take the NCCAOM test and apply for acupuncture licenses in different states. However, some states, such as California, do not accept the NCCAOM test because California has its own test. And New Jersey requires an oral examination besides the NCCAOM test. You can visit your state government's website for details.

2. A second group of non-physician acupuncturists practicing in the United States are those trained in foreign countries. There are many of these acupuncturists currently practicing acupuncture in the U.S. In spite of their different background, their acupuncture schools must all be accredited by the Accreditation Commission for Acupuncture and Oriental Medicine (ACAOM) www.acaom.org/ and all the foreign graduates must take the NCCAOM test in order to apply for the license in most of the states.

When choosing an acupuncturist, check the practitioner's background and interview him or her. To determine the background, you may want to visit the websites of your state government and the ones listed above. You should ask what is involved in the treatment, how likely it is to help your condition, and how much it will cost, and find out if the expense is covered by your insurance.

MY PERSONAL ADVICE

From the above information, you may have learned something about how to select your acupuncturist, but there are many different acupuncture practitioners. So, as an M.D. acupuncturist, here is my own personal advice.

- Check their licenses and background. If the doctor is a physician, how, when, and where did he/she get his/her M.D. license and acupuncture training? If the doctor is a non-physician acupuncturist, does he/she have license? This is the most important question.
- Another important thing in checking credentials is to find out whether or not the practitioner was trained in China, which is considered the gold standard for becoming an effective acupuncturist. It takes a minimum of five years intense training to become certified in China, and the highly skilled practitioners trained in this system have developed a profound understanding of the whole body's reaction to the acupuncture process that can be of great benefit to you.
- Ask for references. A good doctor usually has excellent references.
- Trust your first impression. If you do not feel right, it is better for you to leave.

REACTIONS TO ACUPUNCTURE

Following an acupuncture session, a person's symptoms may become worse, reported Dr. Ruth Kidson. However, that is a good sign. This also occurs in other therapies, such as homeopathy (where it is known as aggravation), and in energy healing (where it is called a healing reaction). This is always a sign that the person is going to respond well to treatment, so it should be an encouragement to continue the therapy. The reaction usually lasts twenty-four hours or less, and is often quickly followed by a considerable improvement in the condition.[2]

"One great advantage of acupuncture and other holistic therapies is that, fairly early on in the treatment, you are likely to start feeling better—possibly even before the symptoms of your disease start to improve," Kidson said. "The ultimate aim of acupuncture is to bring you into perfect balance. It is this balance, and not just an absence of disease, that constitutes good health."

Except in the Far East, little use is made of acupuncture in place of anesthesia, she continued. However, since a number of anesthetists use acupuncture in their pain clinics, it is possible that some might be willing to use it for suitable patients having minor operations. It is possible to have acupuncture in place of painkillers during childbirth, which is advantageous as there are no risks to the baby.

PART TWO

Theories of Traditional Chinese Medicine

8

The Yin and Yang Theory

Yin and yang are philosophical concepts. The theory suggests that every object in the universe consists of two complementary opposites, the negative and the positive, which the Chinese called the yin and the yang, and which are at the same time interdependent and in conflict. This perpetual interplay between yin and yang, where the states of yin and yang must succeed each other, is the universal law of the material world, the principle and source of the existence of a variety of things, as well as the root cause for the flourishing and perishing of things. Life and growth belong to yang, death and storage belong to yin. The surface of the body is yang, the interior is yin, and the same applies to every internal organ.

The inter-opposing, inter-depending, inter-consuming/supporting, and inter-transforming relationships between yin and yang can be summarized as the *unity of opposites* law. Further, these four relationships between yin and yang are interconnected, with each one influencing the other and each being the cause or effect of the others.

All are applied extensively in traditional Chinese medicine to explain the physiology and pathology of the human body, and also serve as a guide to diagnosis and treatment in clinical work.

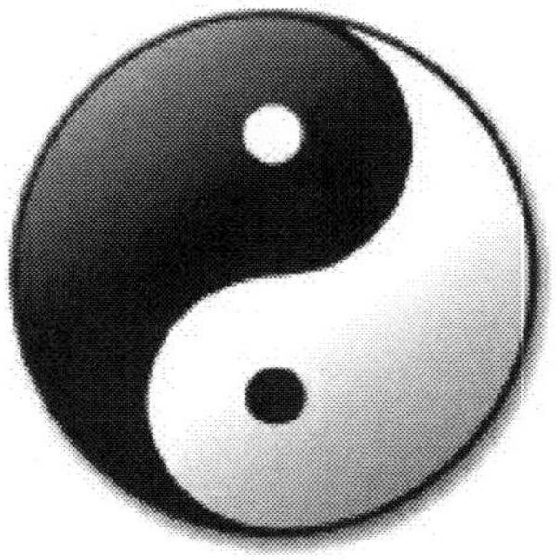

Black is yin, white is yang. Inside the circle, you can see the yin-yang balance represented—yin inside yang, and yang inside yin.

YIN AND YANG

YIN	YANG
Water	Fire
Moon	Sun
Darkness	Lightness
Earth	Heaven
Rest	Activities
West	East
Right	Left
Downward	Upward

THE CHARACTERISTICS OF YIN AND YANG AND THEIR RELATIONSHIP TO EACH OTHER

As shown in the table on the previous page, yin and yang are always are opposite phenomena or objects.

The Opposition of Yin and Yang

Ancient scholars used water and fire to symbolize the basic properties of yin and yang.

The basic properties of yin simulate those of water, including coldness and dampness. Yin represents interior, slow, dark, night, dimness, inhibition, quietness, loss of strength, rest, downward, and interior direction.

The basic properties of yang are like those of fire, including hotness and brightness. Yang represents exterior, quick, light, brightness, day, excitement, movement, and upward, active, outward direction.

These opposites are relative, not absolute; they are in a dynamic balance of many opposing forces. For example, the day is considered yang, the night yin; however, during the daytime, the morning is yang and the afternoon is yin. By the same token, the first half of the night is yin, the second half is yang. Noon and midnight are the turning points, which keep the dynamic balance of the opposing forces.

The Interdependence of Yin and Yang

Yin and yang are both opposite each other *and* mutually dependent. Yin does not exist without yang, and vice versa. For example, if there is no daytime, there will be no nighttime; if there is no concept of dark, there will be no light because they are mutually reliant on each other.

The Mutual Consumption and Support of Yin and Yang

Yin and yang are in a state of continuous mutual consumption and support. For example, follow the sunrise in the morning and yin will gradually decrease. At noontime, yang will be in its strongest and most powerful stage; in the afternoon, however, yang will gradually decrease and yin will start to rise, and by night yang is almost gone and the predominant force is yin. That is true until midnight, when yang gradually starts to increase as yin gradually decreases; by morning, yang is rising again, demonstrating why yin and yang are mutually consuming and supporting.

The Four States of Yin and Yang

- Preponderance of yin. This occurs during the evening before midnight.
- Preponderance of yang. This occurs during the morning in daytime.
- Weakness of yin. This occurs in the morning.
- Weakness of yang. This occurs in the first half of the night.

The Inter-Transformation of Yin and Yang

Yin and yang are two aspects of one mutually dependent phenomenon. Yin can transform to yang; Yang can transform to yin. For instance, summer changes into winter, day changes into night, heat into cold, life into death, even happiness can change into unhappiness.

The Infinite Division of Yin and Yang

Yin and yang are in a constant state of change. Anything in this world can be divided into yin and yang. For example, in the human body, the back of the body is seen as yang and the front as yin. However, the top of the body is yang and the bottom of the body is yin, the left side of the body is yang, and the right side is yin, showing that yin and yang can be divided indefinitely. *This is a very important theory in understanding TCM.*

APPLYING THE YIN AND YANG THEORY TO TRADITIONAL CHINESE MEDICINE (TCM)

The yin-yang theory can be applied to all different aspects of nature as well as to traditional Chinese medicine. TCM applies the yin-yang theory to its clinical concepts, such as the structure of the human body, its physiological function, and the pathological changes that can occur, along with their diagnosis and treatment.

Yin and Yang Theory and the Structure of the Human Body

There are three aspects of yin-yang relative to the structure of the human body.

1. **The anatomic location.** According to TCM theory, the upper body is yang and the lower body is yin; the external body is yang, and the interior body is yin. The medial aspects (towards the midline of the body) of the four extremities are yin, and the lateral aspects (away from the midline of the body) of the four extremities are yang.
2. **TCM applies the yin-yang theory to the internal organ system, separating the organs into two parts.** The organs with active movement, such as the gallbladder, large intestine, small intestine, stomach, and urinary bladder, are yang

organs known as *FU* organs. The organs with imperceptively active movement, such as the heart, kidney, liver, lung, and spleen, are yin organs known as the *Zang* organs. TCM physicians treat their patients using the yin-yang principal. For active yang organs, such as the gallbladder, large intestine, small intestine, stomach, and urinary bladder, treatment is mainly to keep these organs moving. For inactive yin organs, such as the heart, kidney, liver, lung, and spleen, treatment by acupuncture and Chinese herbs is mainly to keep the vital energy of these organs smooth, as yin is inactive and in stasis.

3. **Yin and yang theory is applied to the acupuncture meridian system.** There are yin meridians and yang meridians. Those paired with the yin organs are yin meridians, such as the heart, kidney, liver, lung, and spleen meridians. Those paired with the yang organs are yang meridians, such as the gallbladder, large intestine, small intestine, stomach, and urinary bladder.

Yin-Yang Theory and the Physiological Function of the Human Body

Yang is responsible for all the functional activities of each of the organs. However, their activities are also related to yin because the various nutrients nourishing each of the organs are all substances of yin. Therefore, the yin supports the organ activities of the yang, and the yang depends on the yin nutrients to support them.

Yin-Yang Theory and the Pathological Changes in the Human Body

Traditional Chinese medicine also applies the yin-yang theory to the pathological changes in the human body. For example, the kidney organ has both yang and yin. If the kidney has yang deficiency, the human body will feel cold, and have low energy, poor digestion, and stasis (stoppage of the normal flow of a body substance); if there is a yin kidney deficiency, the person will feel hot and thirsty, will sleep poorly, and have low energy. Since the human body and the organs must keep yin and yang balanced, if there is any one deficiency or excess, it will cause different kinds of problems in each organ.

Yin-Yang Theory and Clinical Diagnosis and Treatment

An imbalance of yin and yang in the organs can cause all the different kinds of pathological changes, and based on these pathological changes, traditional Chinese medicine will make a clear clinical diagnosis. For example, if a person comes in complaining of a stomach ache, the first thing is to find out if this is a yang or yin excess or deficiency. If the stomach has too much fire, it is in yang excess, and the person will have a very strong appetite, a bad taste, a smell in the mouth along with some ulceration, a toothache, etc. If someone has a yang deficiency in the stomach, he or she will also have a mild stomach ache, but may love drinking hot water, pressing the stomach, or using warmth on it.

In each case, the treatments are completely different because the clinical diagnoses are different. One treatment for the yang excess is to purge the fire, the other is to improve the yang component. If there is a yang excess of the stomach, the best treatment is to use Chinese herbs and acupuncture to purge the fire and the excess yang. If there is a deficiency of yang in the stomach, herbs and acupuncture will be used to improve the stomach yang. If there is a yin excess, acupuncture points and Chinese herbs that can intensify yang will be used in order to keep the yin-yang balance. If there is a yin deficiency, acupuncture points and Chinese herbs that can intensify yin will be selected. Both treatments demonstrate how the yin and yang theory can be used as a guide for clinical diagnosis and treatment to improve the stomach yang.

9

The Five Elements Theory

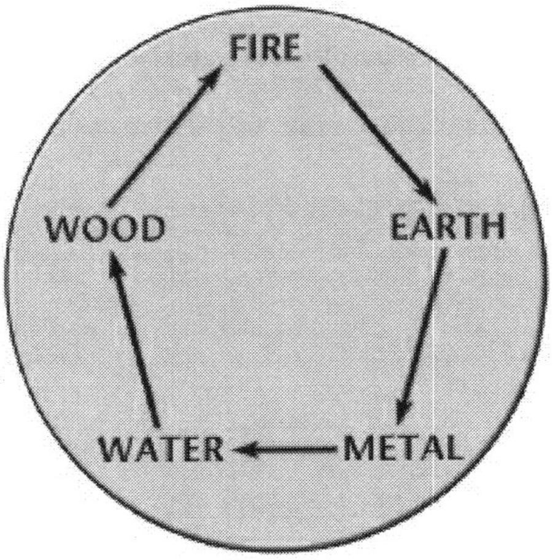

FIGURE 9.1

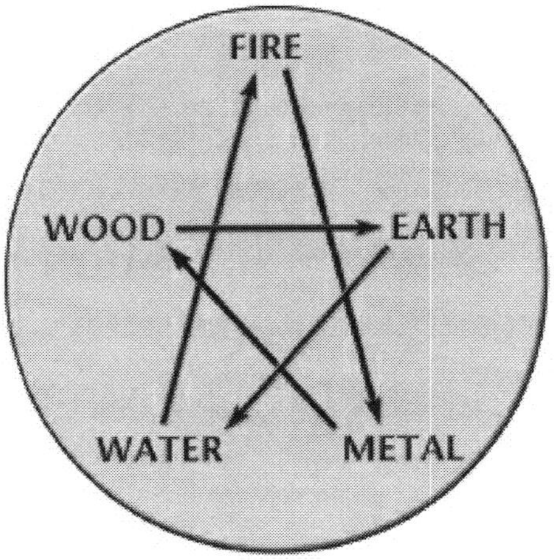

FIGURE 9.2

In traditional Chinese medicine, the Chinese divided the world into five elements (as opposed to four in the West), and everything on earth belonged to one or several of these categories: wood, fire, earth, metal, and water. When the elements of a system are in balance, the cycles of generation and control function to both nourish and contain one another. Based on observation in nature, the ancient TCM practitioners realized these five elements have three different functions and reactions with each other.

- For the first, Figure 9.1 demonstrates what is called the intergeneration function. Specifically, wood will burn to generate a fire; when wood has burned, it generates ashes—earth; from earth, metal is mined, so earth generates metal; if heated, metal becomes liquid, like water; and water is necessary to grow plants and wood, so in effect water generates wood.
- The second function and reaction is interacting and overacting. Wood will inhibit earth, earth will inhibit water, water will inhibit fire, and fire will inhibit metal. According to observations since ancient times, wood can be used as a tool to dig in the earth. Earth can be used to establish a dam to prevent the overflow of water. Water can extinguish fire; fire can dissolve metal; and metal can destroy wood, by cutting it. These are all called interacting and overacting and are demonstrated in Figure 9.2.
- The third function and reaction is counteracting (opposing and mitigating effects by contrary action), and the five elements can also oppose in return (see Figure 9.3). When the elements are

out of balance, when elements grow out of proportion, they overact on one another and bring about mental disharmonies, such as anger, grief, fear, or worry, and physical complaints in the different organ systems. Identifying and treating an element that is out of balance can restore harmony to the body, mind, and spirit.

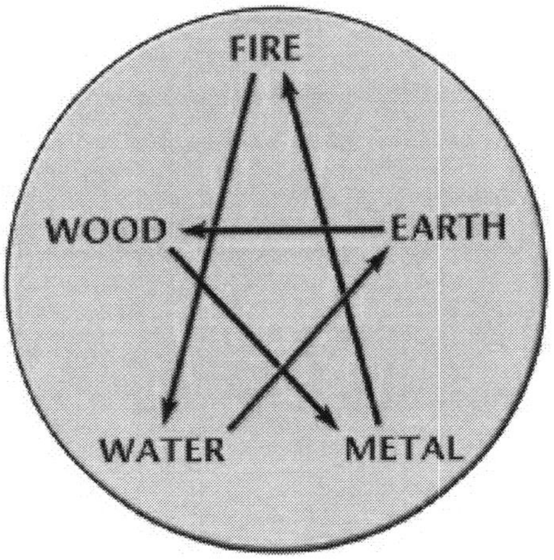

FIGURE 9.3

The counteracting relation of the five elements implies that one of the five elements is so strong that it counteracts another element, which then becomes overacted upon. For instance, on the one hand, wood is normally acted upon by metal. On the other hand, metal may be too weak to act upon wood, but is counteracted upon by wood when it is particularly strong.

The overacting and counteracting relations of the five elements are both abnormal interactions. For instance, when wood is extremely strong, it cannot only overact upon earth, but it can counteract metal;

when metal is extremely weak, it cannot only be counteracted by wood, but it can be overacted upon by fire. Hence, there is a connection between overaction and counteraction. For additional information, go to: www.aworldofgood-health.com/articles/five-elements.htm

Associated with each element is an extensive set of correspondences. For example, wood is associated with anger, the liver meridian, spring, the color green, and the eyes. Water is associated with fear, the kidney meridian, winter, the color black, and the ears. See also: www.balanceflow.com/Rfiveelement.htm

APPLICATION OF FIVE ELEMENTS THEORY TO TRADITIONAL CHINESE MEDICINE

TCM applies these five elements to the organ system. For example, it uses wood to describe the liver because wood always grows and spreads out, which means that the liver's function will always spread out to smoothly extend the liver's energy. If the liver's energy is interfered with, its function will be unsteady because the liver is the organ that controls blood and emotion, and the liver function should be like wood, always growing without any interference. This is when the liver is similar to wood.

TCM uses fire to describe the heart. The heart is just like a fire; it does not have very much yin so the heart acts as a pure yang machine to promote and pump the blood to the entire body through its Yang energy. It needs to work like fire and go upward. Table 9.1 below describes the elements in the organs.

TABLE 9.1

	WOOD	FIRE	EARTH	METAL	WATER
Yin organs	Liver	Heart	Spleen	Lung	Kidney
Yang organs	Gall-bladder	Small intestine	Stomach	Large intestine	Urinary bladder
Sensory organs	Eyes	Tongue	Mouth	Nose	Ears
Emotions	Anger	Joy	Worry	Sadness	Fear
Color	Green	Red	Yellow	White	Black
Tastes	Sour	Bitter	Sweet	Pungent	Salty
Development	Birth	Growth	Transformation	Harvest	Storage

10

The Zang-Fu Organs

THE FIVE ZANG ORGANS

The Heart

The heart has three main functions in the human body.

- *The heart governs the blood* and the blood vessels and manifests itself on the face. The heart functions as a pump, pushing the blood throughout the entire body through the blood vessels. If the heart-pumping function is not strong enough to supply the tissues, the vivid life color under the skin cannot show on the face. Therefore, TCM theory believes the heart dominates the blood vessels which manifest themselves on the face.
- *The heart houses the mind.* The mind, as it is understood, is a broad concept of brain and consciousness and includes vital activities of the whole body. According to TCM theory, the heart houses and controls the mind and the consciousness. Western cultures also believe the heart controls the mind and consciousness. For example, you often hear, "you are out of your mind," which actually means you are confused, or "my heart is broken," which means a person is very sad, etc

- *The heart has an opening into the tongue.* TCM usually observes the tongue to diagnose if someone has anemia, loss of blood, or similar, as the color and shape of the tongue indicate the condition of the heart.

The Liver

- *The liver's main function is storing blood.* It warehouses the blood and it regulates the volume of circulation. When the liver is malfunctioning, there is a blood deficiency and the normal activities of the body will be affected because of this.
- *The liver maintains the free flow of qi.* This is the energy of the human body, which flourishes and supports the functioning of the entire body. Qi is under the control of the liver, and the liver is related to three sub functions.
- *Liver energy.* Liver qi is closely related to emotional activity. When liver qi is stagnated there will be mental depression, paranoia, or even weeping, and when the liver qi is hyperactive, there will be dreams, dizziness, disturbed sleep, insomnia, irrational behaviors, vertigo, and similar.
- *The liver regulates the digestion.* Dysfunction of the liver may affect the secretion and excretion of bile. This causes energy stagnation and will result in poor digestion and appetite. For example, if someone is angry, this person might be too angry to eat because he or she feels full. TCM believes,

therefore, that excessive liver qi (wood) will inhibit the activities of the stomach (earth).

- *The liver is related to pumping the blood* throughout the entire body.
- *The liver controls muscles and tendons,* and its function manifests itself in the nails. The tendons link the joints and muscles and dominate the movement of the extremities. Because the liver nourishes the tendons of the whole body to maintain the function of physiological activities, when the liver's blood is deficient, this nourishment of the tendons will diminish, and this will cause weakness of the tendons, numbness of the limbs, and dysfunction of the joints in contraction and relaxation. Since the liver's blood manifests itself in the nails, if there is a deficiency of liver yin in the blood, the nails will be pale.
- *The liver has an opening in the eye.* If there is a deficiency of liver yin, it will cause dryness of the eye, blurred vision, and sometimes night blindness. If the liver fire is increased, it will cause facial redness, swelling, and painful eyes.

The Spleen

The spleen predominantly helps digestion and controls blood. It has the following functions.

- *Transportation and transformation.* The spleen can transform and transport water in the blood to the four extremities.

- *The spleen can limit the blood inside the blood vessels.* This means that the spleen qi energy has the function of keeping the blood circulating in the blood vessels and preventing the blood from leaking out of the blood vessels.
- *The spleen dominates the muscles and the four extremities.* It can transport and transform the essentials of food and water to nourish the muscles and the four limbs. If the nourishment is inadequate, the muscles of the four limbs will be weak and sot, which will impact the spleen and cause a deficiency.
- *The spleen has an opening into the mouth and manifests itself on the lips.* Its function of transportation and transformation is heavily related to food intake and the sense of taste. When the spleen is functioning normally, there will be a good appetite and a normal sense of taste. If the spleen is malfunctioning, there will be a poor appetite, an impaired sense of taste, such as a sticky sweetish sensation in the mouth. Since the lips are the indicator for the spleen, if the spleen is healthy, there will be ample energy in the blood and the lips will be red and nourished. If the spleen's energy (qi) is deficient, it will lead to a deficiency of qi in the blood and the lips will be pale.

The Lung

The lung is the respiratory organ and its main function is as follows.

- *The lung dominates in two ways.* It dominates the qi (energy) of respiration and it dominates the qi of the whole body.
- *The lung dominates skin and hair.* The lung can distribute the energy, such as defensive qi, which originates from the lung and spreads out to the body surface to protect the entire body, and circulates body fluid to the entire body to warm and moisten the muscles, skin, and hair. The skin and hair located on the surface of the body must depend on the lung's distributing function, so the lung is paramount in dispersing skin and hair; and vice versa, the skin and hair are surface indicators that are paramount in the lung's function.
- *The lung also dominates the body's descending fluids and regulates the water passages.* The lungs are located at the top of the body, therefore, the lung's qi descends to promote circulation of qi and fluid throughout the body and to direct the qi and fluid downwards. If there is a dysfunction of the lung, if the lung's energy is unable to spread out and descend throughout the entire body, its energy will be handicapped, causing coughs, shortness of breath, or other respiratory problems.

- *The lung has an opening into the nose, which is the pathway for respiration.* The respiratory and olfactory functions depend on lung qi.

The Kidneys

The kidneys are the power energy of the body and they have the following functions.

- *Storing nutritional essentials and dominating development and reproduction.* The kidney stores the essential substance of food transported by the spleen and stomach, and also the congenital substances and essences transported and inherited from parents. All these are stored in the kidney. The kidney also affects the body's reproduction and development, which completely relies on the kidney qi.
- *The kidney also dominates water metabolism.* It can redistribute the water and the waste material, which will go out through the urine by the function of kidney qi.
- *The kidney controls the reception of qi.* It can control the qi transportation from the lung, spleen, stomach, and liver, so the passage of qi in the lung will be active, and the stomach and spleen qi will be functional only when the kidney qi is strong.
- *The kidney can produce bone marrow* and, in turn, control bone density.
- *The kidney has an opening into the ears.* When the kidney qi is deficient, as for example when

people age, their hearing will gradually diminish. This is because of kidney deficiency.

- *A kidney deficiency manifests itself in the hair* because the hair relies on the nourishment of the kidney essence to grow. If there is a kidney deficiency, such as can be found in older people, the hair will become gray and even white.

The Pericardium

The pericardium is a membrane surrounding the heart. When pathological qi invades the heart, the pericardium is always the first to be attacked and this invasion of the pericardium by pathological qi will often affect the normal function of the heart. Therefore TCM believes that the pericardium is the protector of the heart.

THE SIX FU ORGANS

The Gallbladder

The gallbladder's major function is to store and excrete bile. It controls judgment and controls thoughts, such as dreams, fears, etc.

The Stomach

The stomach controls digestion.

The Small Intestine

The main function of the small intestine is to absorb and digest food. It also separates unwanted food particles from the essence of the food.

The Large Intestine

The large intestine is the transportation organ. Its main function is to absorb water and turn the food remainder into feces to be excreted.

The Urinary Bladder

The urinary bladder's function is to store fluid and excrete urine.

San Jiao

San Jiao has many functions, but it is a not a clearly understood organ. Its main function is to host and separate the function of the upper, middle, and lower three parts of the organs along the chest and abdominal cavities.

11

The Meridians

There are fourteen major meridians in traditional Chinese medicine. The main function of the fourteen meridians is to produce, store, and activate the interior and exterior distribution of qi energy and blood across the body. Based on the yin-yang and organ theories, there are twelve regular meridians, six on each side of the body, with two more running up the middle of the body. The twelve major meridians are considered the basis of all theory and treatment, and each one corresponds to, and is named for, the organ system with which it is associated.

THE SIX PAIRS OF MERIDIANS

- Lung and large intestine meridians
- Stomach and spleen meridians
- Heart and small intestine meridians
- Urinary bladder and kidney meridians
- Pericardium and San Jiao meridians
- Gallbladder and liver meridians

In addition to the six pairs, there are other two very important meridians, Du and Ren. Du is located in the midline of the body's back, Ren is located in the midline of the frontal body. These meridians do not belong to the twelve regular meridians, but they have the very important function of implementing the input of the internal organs to the entire body.

All the meridians form a network of pathways, or channels, along which the qi energy flows. Each meridian has its own organ, such as the lung, through which it passes to receive qi energy from the source.

THE FUNCTIONS OF THE FOURTEEN MERIDIANS

- They carry and transport qi and blood and regulate yin and yang. Under normal circumstances, the system of the meridians functions as transport to carry qi and blood and regulate the balance between the yin and yang of the whole body.
- They resist and prevent the invasion of pathogens. If there are symptoms and signs of pathological conditions, the meridians will reflect these.
- They also transmit the sensation of the acupuncture needle and regulate conditions of deficiency or excess.

HOW THE MERIDIANS ARE LABELED

The meridians are named for the internal organ with which they are associated, such as the lung meridian. Each meridian has a different number of points. These acupuncture points can be used to adjust the meridian's function, eliminate the pathogenic invasion that is blocking the flow of qi energy, and balance the yin and yang of each organ. There are about 400 acupuncture points along the fourteen major meridians, and approximately fifty acupuncture points which are not regularly located along the fourteen major meridians, and are known as Extraordinary Points. All these acupuncture points have their own names. However, because it is too difficult to remember approximately 450 Chinese names, the W.H.O. is now trying to standardize the names with numbers.

PATHWAYS OF THE FOURTEEN MAIN MERIDIANS

The Lung Meridian

The lung meridian starts from the region of the abdomen (San Jiao) and runs down to connect to the large intestine. It then ascends to the stomach, travels through the diaphragm and heart and enters the lung; it passes through the respiratory tract and then ascends to the throat and emerges at Lu 1 Zhong Fu. From there, it descends along the arm until it reaches the radius, i.e. the lateral side of the forearm, goes to the wrist and ends at the tip of the thumb at Lu 11, Shao Shang, and connects to the large intestine meridian. (See Figure 11.1 on the following page.)

TABLE 11.1. INTRODUCTION TO THE NAMING REGULATIONS AND ABBREVIATIONS

No.	NAME	ABBREV.	START POINT	END POINT
1	Lung	Lu	Lu 1	Lu 11
2	Large Intestine	LI	LI 1	LI 20
3	Stomach	St	St 1	St 45

No.	NAME	ABBREV.	START POINT	END POINT
4	Spleen	Sp	Sp 1	Sp 21
5	Heart	Ht	Ht 1	Ht 9
6	Small Intestine	SI	SI 1	SI 19
7	Urinary Bladder	UB	UB 1	UB 67
8	Kidney	Ki	Ki 1	Ki 27
9	Pericardium	PC	Pc 1	PC 9
10	San Jiao	SJ	SJ 1	SJ 23
11	Gallbladder	Gb	Gb 1	Gb 44
12	Liver	Li	Li 1	Li 14
13	Du	Du	Du 1	Du 28
14	Ren	Ren	Ren 1	Ren 24

The Large Intestine Meridian

The large intestine meridian originates from the inside tip of the index finger (the second finger). It then travels along the index finger at LI 4 He Gu, between the tendons and muscles at the wrist, and up the arm. It then reaches the shoulder at the point of LI 15 Jian Yu, and from LI 15 it connects to the Du 14 Da Zhui (the connecting point of 6 yang meridians) and then descends to the lung. At the St 12 Que Pen it meets with the lung, and ascends to the cheek and enters the gums at the lower teeth. It then crosses over the cheek to end at the site of nose at LI 20 Yin Xiang, where it links with the stomach meridian. (See Figure 11.2.)

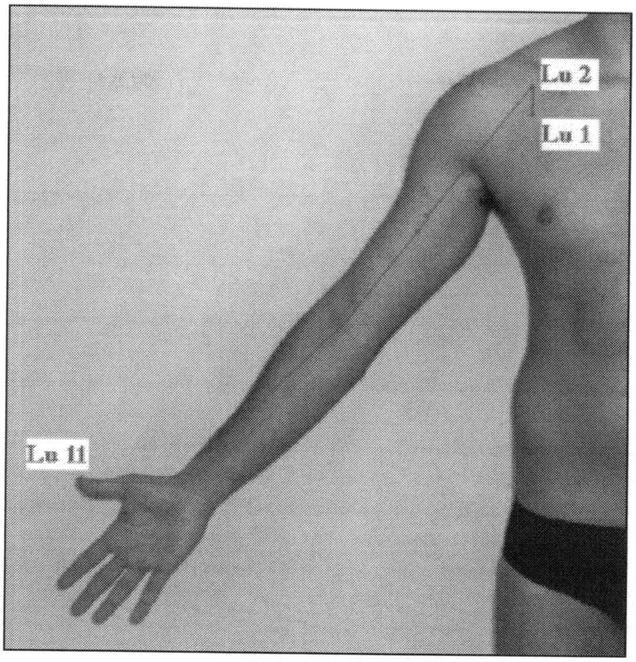

FIGURE 11.1

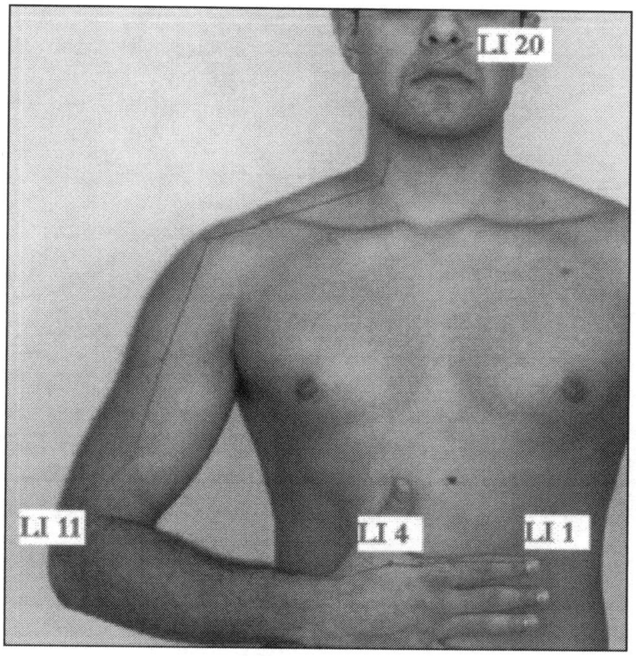

FIGURE 11.2

The Stomach Meridian

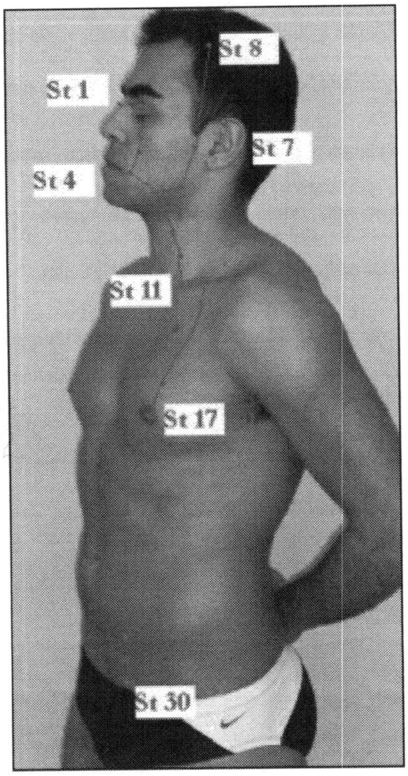

FIGURE 11.3

The stomach meridian begins at the side of the nose, Li 20 Yin Xiang, then ascends along the nose and meets the Urinary Bladder meridian at UB 1 Jing Ming (see Figure 11.10). It then descends parallel to the nose, penetrates the jaw and enters the upper gums. It curves around the lips and links with the Ren Meridian at Ren 24 Cheng Jiang in the groove of the chin. It then runs along the lower jaw and extends in front of the ear to reach the forehead.

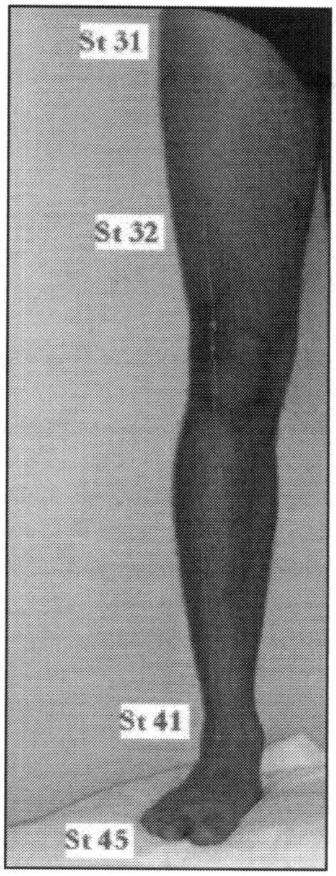

FIGURE 11.4

From the stomach, St 5 Da Yin, a branch goes down to the throat to the St 9 Ren Yin, and continues down to travel though the diaphragm, entering the stomach and the spleen.

From the stomach, St 5 Da Yin, a branch goes down to the throat to the St 9 Ren Yin, and continues down to travel though the diaphragm, entering the stomach and the spleen.

The Spleen Meridian

The spleen meridian starts from the tip of the big toe and runs along the foot to ascend to the tibia. Here, it crosses and runs to the liver meridian,

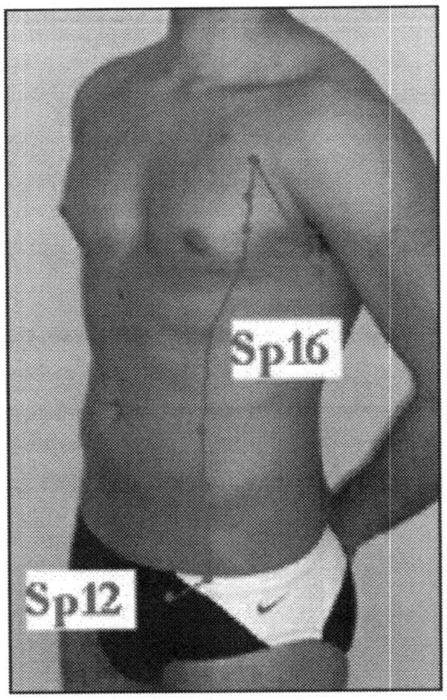

FIGURE 11.5

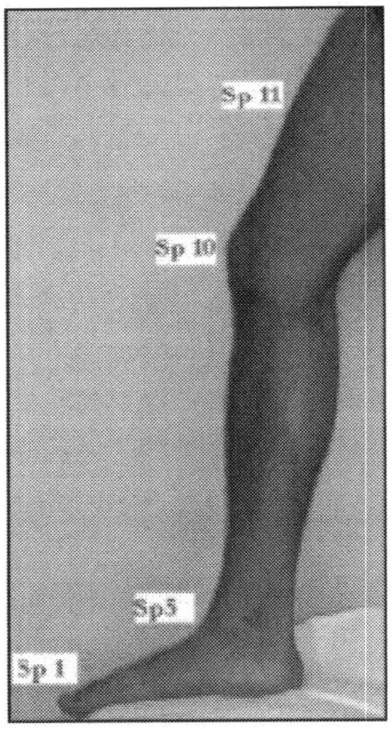

FIGURE 11.6

passes the knee and thigh to enter the abdomen and intersect with Ren 3 Zhong Ji, and Ren 4 Guang Yuan. It then enters the spleen and stomach from where it ascends, traversing the diaphragm to reach the esophagus and cross Lu1 Zhong Fu. It ends at the center of the tongue. From the stomach, a branch goes through the diaphragm and links with the heart. (See Figures 11.5 and 11.6.)

The Heart Meridian

The heart meridian originates in the heart. It then passes through the diaphragm and connects with the small intestine. A branch from the heart ascends to the throat and eye. Another branch from the heart enters the lung and joins the meridian running along the arm to end at the tip of the little finger. (See Figure 11.7.)

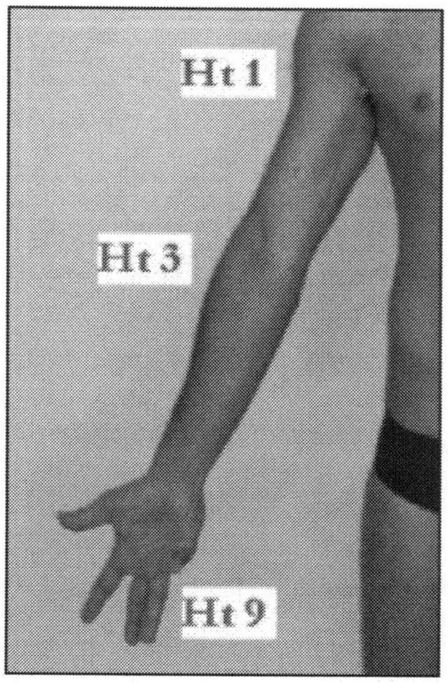

FIGURE 11.7

The Small Intestine Meridian

The small intestine meridian starts at the tip of the little finger follows the hand to the wrist, then ascends along the arm to the shoulder joint, connects

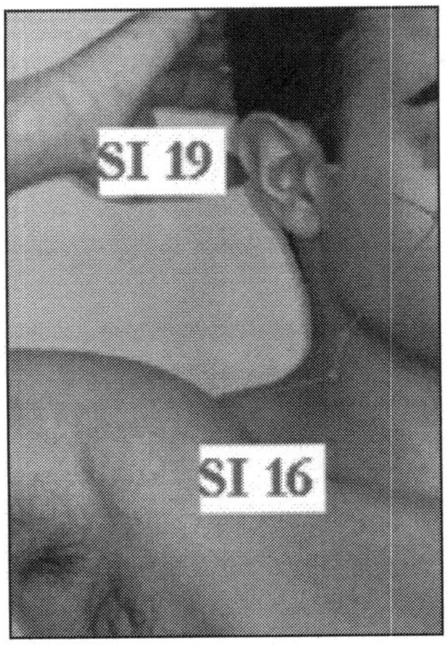

FIGURE 11.8

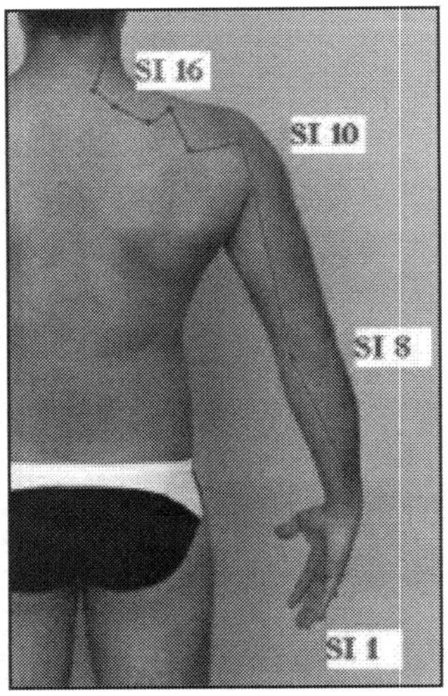

FIGURE 11.9

with Du 14 Da Zhui, and goes forward to St 12 Que Pen to connect to the heart. From the heart, it descends to the esophagus and connects with the small intestine. The pathway of the meridian ascends to the neck and the cheek, and through the cheek to enter the ear. From the cheek, a branch goes to link with the bladder meridian at the inner corner of the eye, BL 1 Jing Ming. (See Figures 11.8 and 11.9.)

The Urinary Bladder Meridian

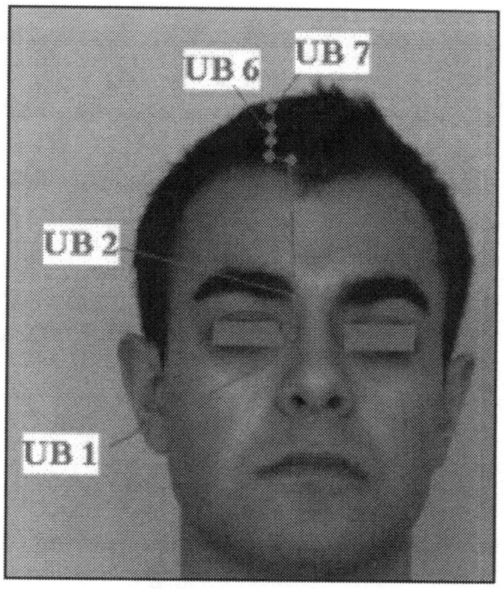

FIGURE 11.10

The bladder meridian starts at the inner eye. It ascends the forehead and joins the Du meridian at Du 20 Bai Hui; from here a branch goes to the temporal area just above the ear. The UB meridian enters the brain to reemerge at the nape of the neck and the muscles of the scapula, meeting the Du meridian at DU 14 Da Zhui. From here, it flows all the way down the back from the lumbar area of the spine where it enters the kidney and bladder. Another branch from the eye runs down the back to the scapula, down the back to the gluteus muscles, where it meets the previous branch and runs along the back to end at the fifth toe at UB 67 Zhi Yin to link with the kidney meridian. (See Figures 11.10 and 11.11 on the next page.)

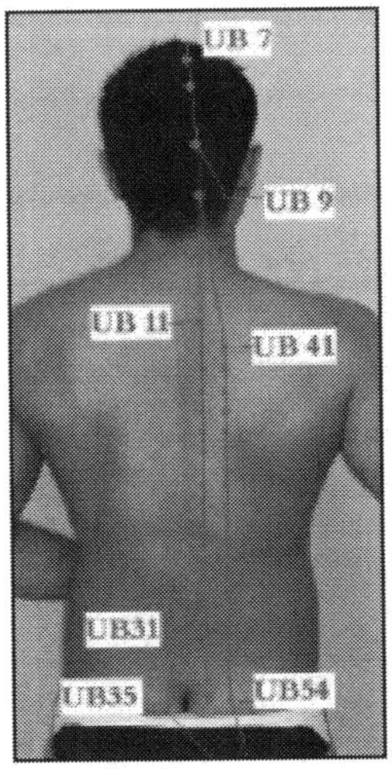

FIGURE 11.11

The Kidney Meridian

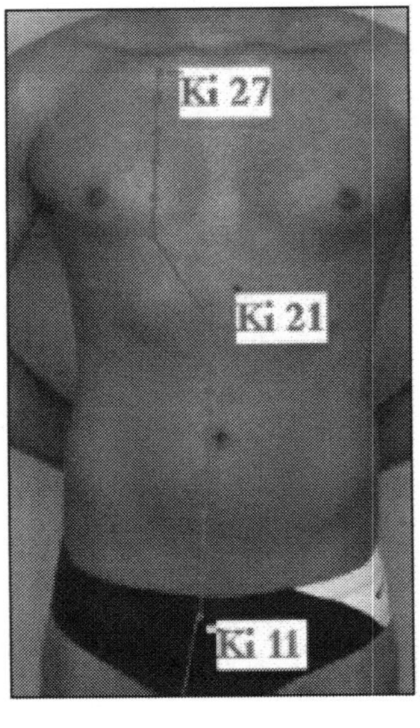

FIGURE 11.12

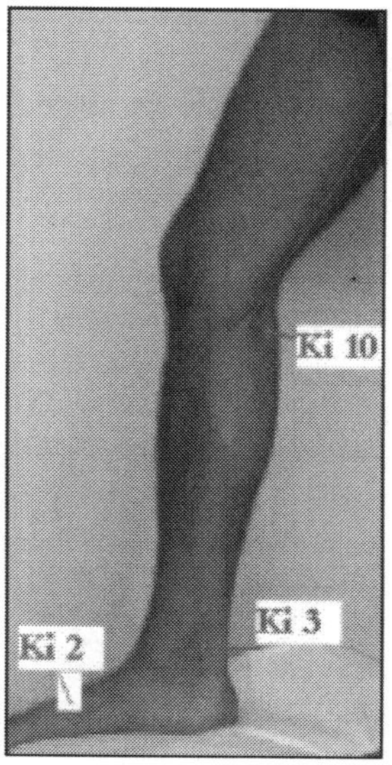

FIGURE 11.13

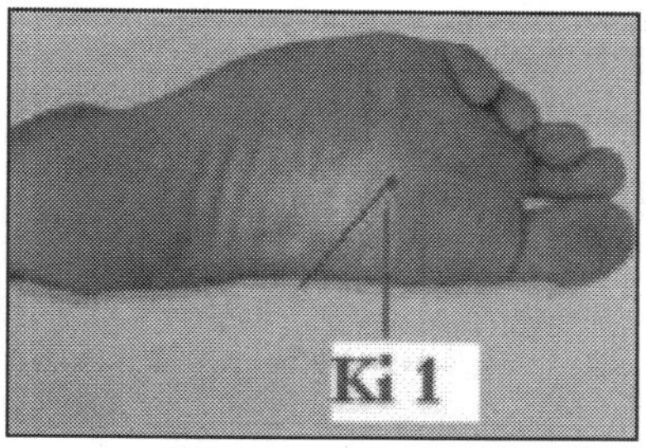

FIGURE 11.14

The kidney meridian starts under the fifth toe and runs to the sole of the foot, Ki 1 Yong Quan, then ascends the leg and intersects with the spleen meridian at Sp 6 San Yin Jiao and travels up to the thigh. It then goes towards the sacrum at Du 1 Chang Qiang, ascends along the lumbar spine and enters the kidney and urinary bladder. A branch leaves the kidney and urinary bladder, then enters the liver, passes through the diaphragm and enters the lung. From here it ascends to the throat and terminates at the root of the tongue. From the lung, another branch joins the heart and flows to the chest to connect with the pericardium meridian. (See Figures 11.12–11.14.)

The Pericardium Meridian

The pericardium meridian originates from the chest and enters the pericardium. It then descends through the diaphragm to the abdomen to communicate with the upper, middle, and lower burner, San Jiao. A branch runs out horizontally from the center of the chest and emerges from the nipple to run down the arm to end at the tip of the middle finger. A branch from point of PC 8 Lao Gong connects with the San Jiao meridian at the point of SJ 1, Guang Chong. (See Figure 11.15.)

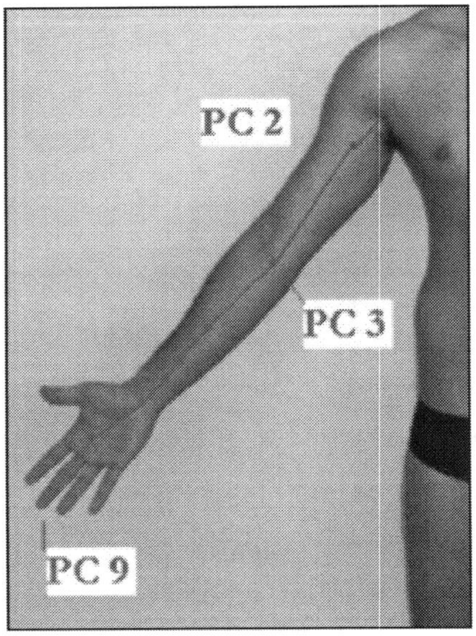

FIGURE 11.15

The San Jiao Meridian

The San Jiao meridian starts at the tip of the ring finger. It flows to the wrist and up the arm and reaches the shoulder joint where it goes down the chest to connect with the precardium. It then descends through the diaphragm to the abdomen to join the middle and lower San Jiao. From the chest at Ren 17 Tan Zhong, a branch ascends to the neck and the region behind the ear to intersect with the gallbladder meridian at GB 6. It then turns downward to the cheek and terminates in the orbit region with small intestine meridian 1. From behind the ear, a branch enters the ear, reemerges in front of the ear and links with the gallbladder meridian. (See Figure 11.16.)

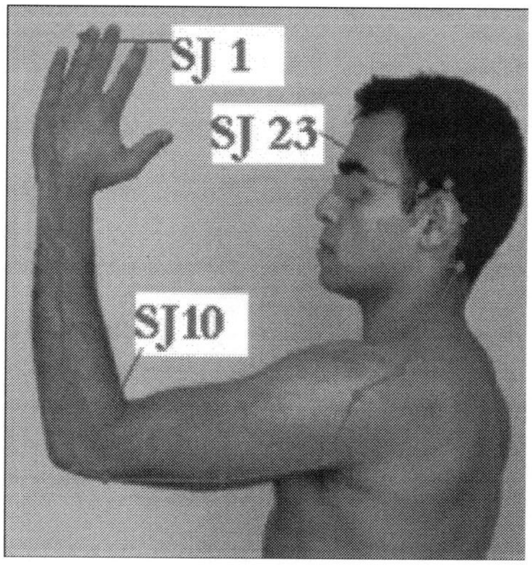

FIGURE 11.16

The Gallbladder Meridian

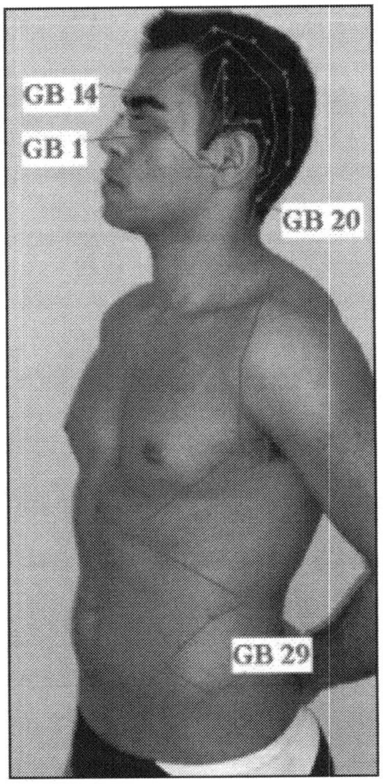

FIGURE 11.17

The gallbladder meridian starts at the eyes. It ascends the forehead where it intersects with the stomach meridian at St 8 Tou Wei, and curves downwards to the region behind the ear at gallbladder 20 Feng Chi; from there it runs down the neck to the clavicle. A branch from the region behind the ear enters the ear to reemerge in front of it and then intersects with the San Jiao meridian at SJ 17 Yi Feng; it then it enters the ear and reemerges in front of the ear to connect SI 19 Ting Gong; another branch flows out from the corner of the eye and meets the San Jiao Meridian in the orbital region. It then descends to the neck and clavicle where it meets the main branch, and from there it descends to the chest and passes through the diaphragm. It enters the liver and gallbladder, then runs down the lateral side of the abdomen to reach the point of gallbladder 30 Huan Tiao.

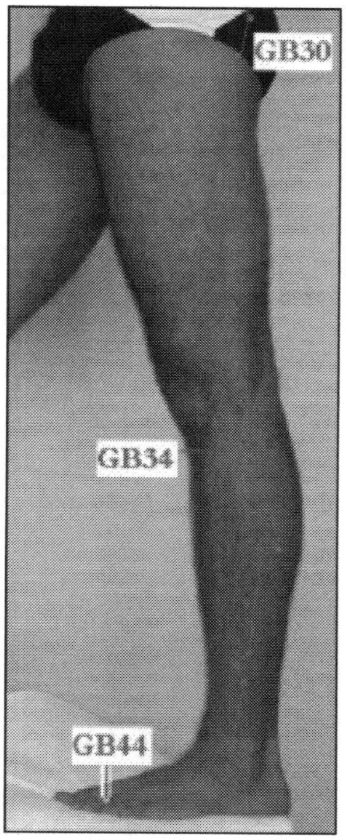

FIGURE 11.18

The main portion of the meridian from the clavicle goes to the lateral side of the chest and then the ribs and hip where it meets the previous branch. It then descends along the thigh and leg to end at the fourth toe.

From the gallbladder 41 Zu Lin Qi, a branch goes to liver 1 Da Dun. (See Figures 11.17 and 11.18.)

The Liver Meridian

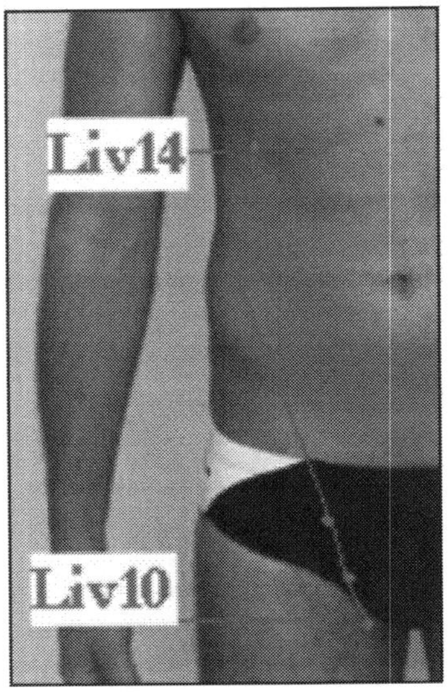

FIGURE 11.19

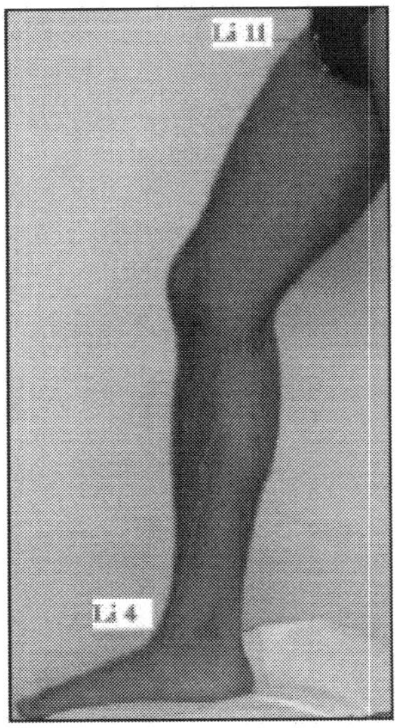

FIGURE 11.20

The liver meridian starts on the big toe and runs upwards on the foot and the leg to connect with Sp 6 San Yin Jiao; It continues up and reaches the genital region, curves around the genitalia, and goes up to the lower abdomen. Proceeding further up, it curves around the stomach and enters the liver and gallbladder. It then continues to ascend, passes through the diaphragm, and branches out in the side ribs; from here it ascends to the throat and reaches the eye. Running further upwards, it goes to the top of the head to meet the Ren meridian. (See Figures 11.19, 11.20, and 11.21.)

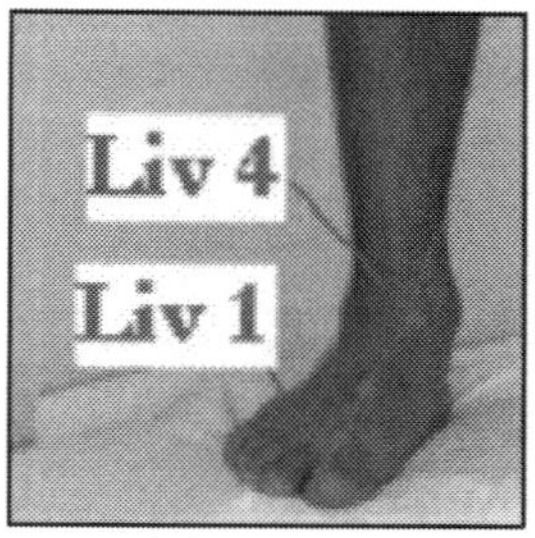

FIGURE 11.21

THE REN AND DU MERIDIANS

The previous twenty-one illustrations portray the regular meridians. There are, however, two other, very important, meridians connected to the twelve regular meridians. They are the Ren meridian and the Du meridian.

Ren Meridian

The Ren meridian originates from the uterus in women, or deep in the lower abdomen or pelvic area in men, and emerges at the perineum Ren 1 Hui Yin. It runs behind the pubic region and all the way up to the throat along the middle line of the body; from the throat it ascends to curve around the lips and up to the eyes to meet the stomach meridian at the point of Stomach 1 Chen Qi. (See Figures 11.22 and 11.23.)

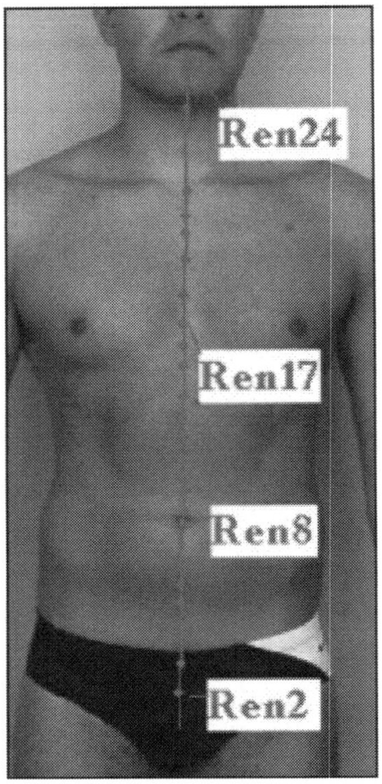

FIGURE 11.22

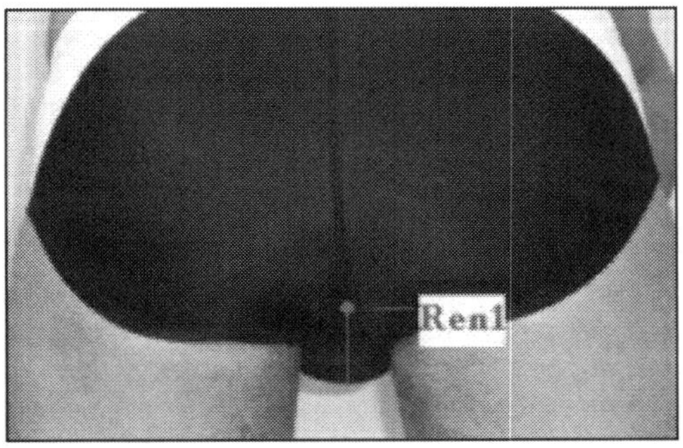

FIGURE 11.23

The Du Meridian

The Du meridian begins in the uterus in women or deep inside the lower abdomen or pelvic area in men and goes to the perineum where it emerges and ascends up the middle line of the back and neck to Du 16 Feng Fu, from where it enters the brain. It then ascends to the front of the face and the upper lip. (See Figures 11.24, 11.25, 11.26, and 11.27.)

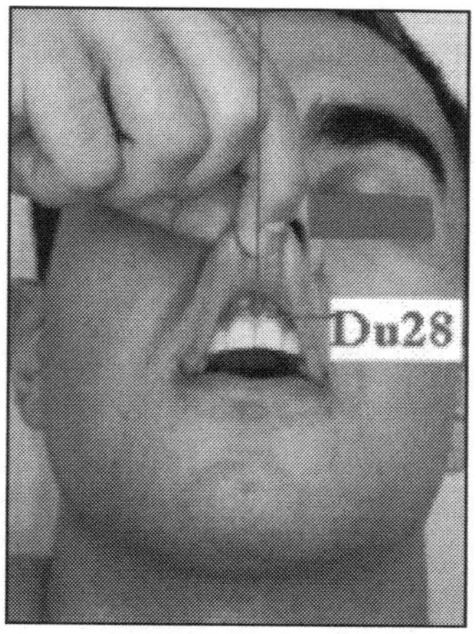

FIGURE 11.24

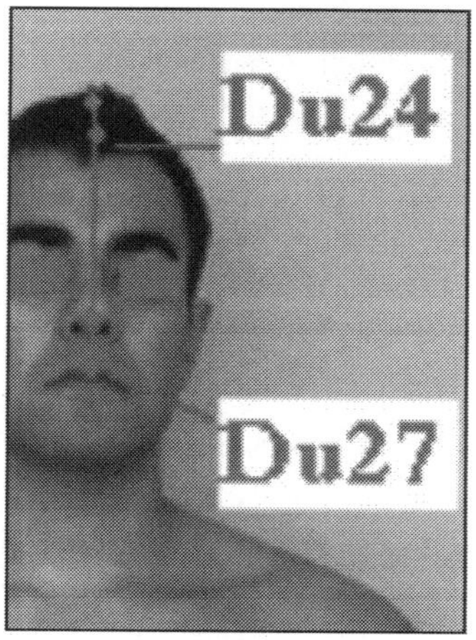

FIGURE 11.25

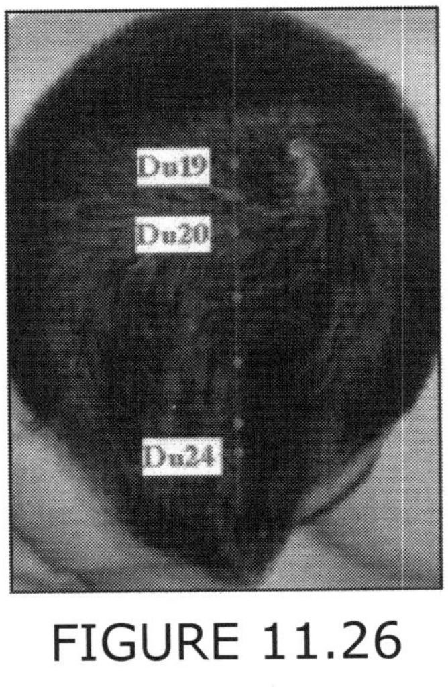

FIGURE 11.26

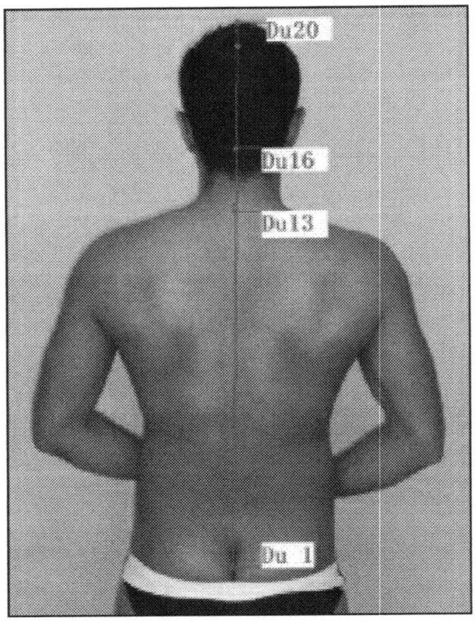

FIGURE 11.27

PART THREE

Case Histories

12

The Common Cold

GEORGIANNE'S COMMON COLD

Georgianne S. is a thirty-seven-year-old woman who works in an office with an air conditioner right next to her desk. One day she began sneezing and complained of a runny nose, nasal obstruction, whitish phlegm, and a sore and scratchy throat, as well as a cough with hoarseness. She also had mild general symptoms like a headache, low-grade fever, and chills. After not feeling well for several days, she called her office to say she was sick and unable to go to work. She then called her primary care physician (PCP), who told her to drink fluids, take some Tylenol, and stay home for about two days, after which she could probably go back to work.

After calling her PCP, Georgianne visited me. She complained of a severe headache and an aching throughout her entire body, especially in her joints, fatigue, poor appetite, difficulty concentrating, and trouble sleeping. Her temperature was 99.8F, her lungs were clear, she had weak and floating pulses, and a smooth, white, tongue coating.

It was most likely that Georgianne had a common cold, an illness caused by a viral infection located in the respiratory tracts—the nose, sinuses, and bronchial tubes. A common cold may last an average of one week, a mild cold may last only two to three days, whereas a severe cold may last for up to two weeks. Often, colds are mixed with influenza, which typically causes fever, muscle ache, and a more severe cough, so people can be confused about the difference between the symptoms of colds and influenza.

WESTERN TREATMENT OF THE COMMON COLD

Traditionally, Western medicine treats the common cold with the following medications.

- Antihistamines. This is the first choice to decrease runny nose, phlegm, etc.
- Non-steroidal anti-inflammatory drugs, such as Tylenol, Advil, etc., to lower temperature and pain.
- Decongestants, which are vasoconstrictors, to decrease secretion.
- Cough suppressants, such as narcotics, to decrease a cough.
- Anticholenergics, to possibly help decrease the runny nose and phlegm.

These medications cannot usually cure the common cold because they are just symptomatic treatments.

Since the cause of the common cold cannot be eradicated by Western medicine, cold symptoms usually last for about one week. However, by using traditional Chinese medicine, it is possible to find a way to eradicate the infection and alleviate the symptoms sooner.

TCM TREATMENT OF THE COMMON COLD

Adults usually experience an average of two to three colds per year. Children, depending on their age and exposure, usually get six to ten. Their noses are the major source of cold viruses, and they usually contract these colds at school.

There are over 100 different cold viruses. Rhinoviruses, which tend to remain in the upper respiratory tract because they cannot reproduce in the warmer parts of the body, are the most important as they cause at least 50 percent of all colds.

According to Chinese medicine, the common cold comes with headaches, nasal obstructions, aversion to wind, and fever. A person with a cold is very sensitive to wind and fever, and Chinese medicine believes it results from the lowered resistance of the body's immune system and the invasion of disease factors.

The main reason for the common cold is that the normal functioning of the immune system has decreased. You often see that, in the same office or the same school, some people get colds, fever, and muscle aches three or four times a year, while others in the same space never catch a cold. Although both groups are exposed to the same virus, one group gets colds and the other does not because of a difference in the functioning of their immune systems.

According to traditional Chinese medicine, there are two types of reasons for the common cold.

- **Wind cold.** This type is usually seasonal, occurring during winter or early spring. At these times, the temperature outside is still cold, and the wind follows the coldness, invading peoples' bodies to cause the symptoms. The main symptoms are chills, low fever, headaches, soreness, pain of the limbs, nasal obstruction, running nose, itching of the throat, cough, hoarse voice, profusely thin sputum, and thin white tongue coating, with a superficial and tense pulse.
- **Wind heat.** The main manifestation of wind heat is fever, sweating, slight sensitivity to wind, pain, a distending sensation of the head, cough with yellow thick sputum, congested sinuses, sore throat, thirst, thin white or yellowish tongue coating, and a superficial and rapid pulse. Usually wind heat occurs in summer and autumn. The weather during these seasons is hot, plus the wind is strong. However, human skin is always perspiring; it contains numerous

tiny holes for the skin to breathe, making the body susceptible to external germs, which can invade the body with wind and heat.

TCM Herbal Formulas for Wind Cold and Wind Heat

Here is a simple, effective formula of Chinese herbs for wind cold.

- Boil red sugar, scallions, fermented soy beans, and ginger for 20 minutes. Drink it after the liquid becomes lukewarm. Be sure to keep your body warm—lie in bed and cover yourself with a comforter, waiting to perspire. Profuse sweating usually occurs overnight and makes the symptoms much less severe than before. This simple concoction often alleviates the wind cold.

Here is a formula for wind heat symptoms.

- Boil onions, scallions, honeysuckle, farsythio (fructus forsythiae), and sugar together and cool before drinking. This mixture is often a sufficient treatment for wind heat.

Acupuncture Treatments for Wind Cold and Wind Heat

For acupuncture treatments, the following points are used.

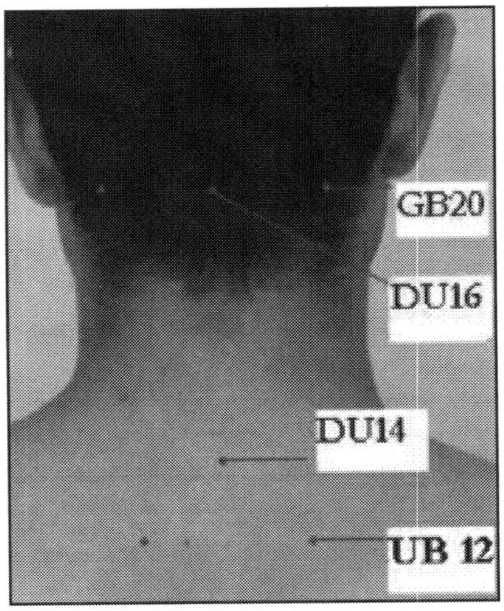

FIGURE 12.1

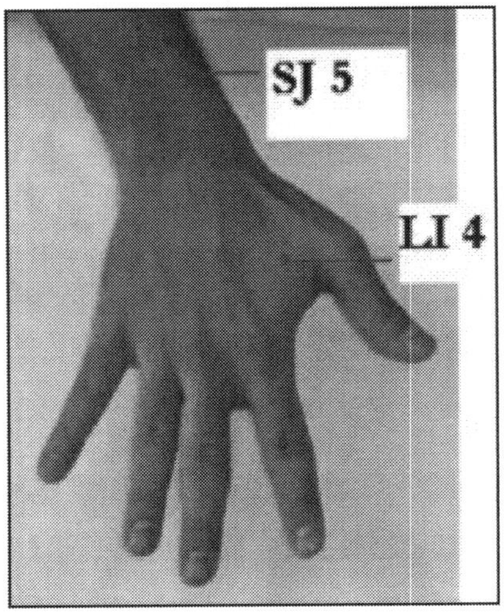

FIGURE 12.2

Wind Cold

Du 16 can be used to eliminate the wind cold and relieve headaches. UB 12 Feng Men, one point of the Urinary Bladder meridian, dominates the surface of the whole body and could regulate the circulation of qi (energy) in the meridian to eliminate the wind cold and relieve chills and fever. Lung 7 Lie Que is the lower point of the lung meridian. It is used to promote the functions of the lung and to help stop coughing. GB 20 Feng Chi assists UB 12 Feng Men to eliminate the wind cold. The rest points are powerful points to eliminate the disease factors of wind cold.

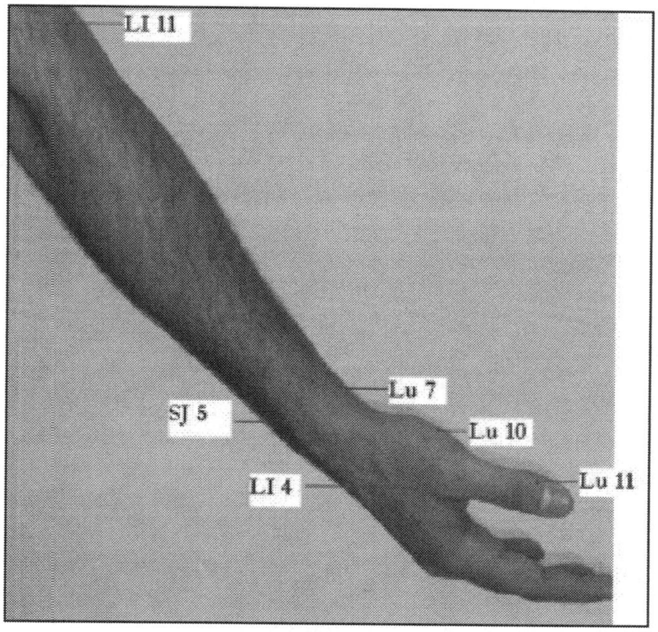

FIGURE 12.3

TABLE 12.1

POINTS	MERIDIAN NUMBER	CONDITIONS HELPED
1 Feng Fu	Du Point 16. See Figure 12.1	Headaches, neck rigidity, blurred vision, sore throat, mental disorders
2 Feng Men	Urinary Bladder Point UB 12. See Figure 12.1	Common cold, cough, fever and headaches, neck rigidity, backache
3 Feng Chi	Gallbladder Point GB 20. See Figure 12.1	Headaches, vertigo, insomnia, pain and stiffness of the neck, blurred vision, glaucoma, red and painful eyes, tinnitus, convulsion, epilepsy, infantile convulsion, common cold, nasal obstruction

POINTS	MERIDIAN NUMBER	CONDITIONS HELPED
4 Lie Que	Lung Point Lu 7. See Figure 12.1	Cough, pain in the chest, asthma, sore throat, spasmodic pain of the elbow and arm
5 He Gu	Large Intestine Point 4. See Figure 12.2	Headaches, pain in the neck, redness swelling and pain of the eye, nosebleed, nasal obstruction, toothache, deafness, swelling of the face, sore throat, facial paralysis, abdominal pain, dysentery, constipation, delayed labor, infantile convulsion, pain, weakness and motor impairment of the upper limbs

Please refer to the accompanying Figures (illustrations) for the locations of the points. And please note that these illustrations are for information only and may not show all the exact locations of the acupuncture points.

Wind Heat

TABLE 12.2

POINTS	MERIDIAN NUMBER	CONDITIONS HELPED
1 Da Zhui	Du 14. See Figure 12.1	Neck pain and rigidity, malaria, epilepsy, afternoon fever, cough, asthma, common cold, back stiffness
2 Qu Chi	LI (Large Intestine) 1 I. See Figure 12.2	Sore throat, toothache, redness and pain in the eye, motor impairment of the upper extremities, abdominal pain, vomiting, diarrhea
3 Wai Guan	San Jiao 5. See Figure 12.3	Headaches, pain in the cheek, strained neck, deafness, tinnitus, motor impairment of the elbow and arm, pain of the fingers, hand tremor
4 He Gu	LI 4. See Figure 12.3	See Table 12.1

POINTS	MERIDIAN NUMBER	CONDITIONS HELPED
5 Yu Ji	Lu (Lung) 10. See Figure 12.2	Cough, sore throat, loss of voice, fever, feverish sensation in the palm
6 Shao Shang	Lu 11. See Figure 12.2	Sore throat, cough, asthma, fever, loss of consciousness, spasmodic pain of the thumb

Please refer to the accompanying Figures (illustrations) for the locations of the points. And please note that these illustrations are for information only and may not show all the exact locations of the acupuncture points.

Da Zhui Du 14 and Qu Qi LI 11 are well known for lowering temperature, and Wai Guan SJ 5, He Gu LI 4, Yu Ji L 10, and Shao Shang L 11 are coordinated to cure pain all over the body and head.

GEORGIANNE'S TREATMENT

Georgianne was diagnosed with wind cold. The acupuncture points Du 16, UB 12, GB 20, L 7, and LI 4 were given and she was also advised to drink ginger and sugar water. Ater two days, she felt much better and was able to return to work.

ACUPRESSURE TIPS FOR WIND COLD AND WIND HEAT FOR USE AT HOME OR OFFICE

Wind Cold

- Press Du 16 and GB 20 with your thumb for about 5 minutes each, and then press LI 4 and

Lu 7 for 5 minutes each. Alternate the points for about 2 sessions.

- Drink the wind cold formula immediately.
- Repeat the sessions with the above points. You should feel better overnight.

Wind Heat

- Press Du 14 and SJ 5 with your thumb for about 5 minutes each, then press LI 4 and Lung 10 for 5 minutes each. Alternate above points for about 2 sessions.
- Drink the wind heat formula immediately.
- Repeat the sessions with the above points. You should feel better overnight.

13

Bronchitis

SUSAN'S BRONCHITIS

Susan W., a forty-five-year-old female, came to my office complaining of a severe cough which had lasted about three or four weeks. It caused tremendous pain in her chest and abdominal muscles and she also coughed out yellowish-greenish phlegm and sometimes experienced wheezing and shortness of breath. She ran a low fever and had chills, muscle aches, nasal congestion, a sore throat, and difficulty swallowing food. Her ears were blocked, making it difficult to hear, and she was extremely uncomfortable in many areas when she came to me for evaluation and treatment.

After a physical examination, I determined that Susan, who looked very tired and was breathing rapidly and noisily, had a low grade fever, a rapid heart rate, nasal congestion, sinus tenderness, and redness in the throat. Examination of the chest with a stethoscope revealed coarse breathing sounds and wheezing. I determined that Susan most likely had bronchitis, an irritation and inflammation of the airways often triggered by an upper respiratory tract infection, such as the common cold or influenza. It can also be caused by a sinus infection, as well as exposure to irritating fumes or dust, fur from cats or dogs, or tobacco smoke.

Bronchitis is an inflammation of the mucous membrane that lines the air passages of the upper airways. The trachea, large airways (bronchi), and small airways (bronchioles) can be involved. There may be swelling and tenderness of the membranes, coughing (with or without sputum production), and reduced airflow. Bronchitis is most commonly caused by a virus, such as influenza, respiratory syncytial virus (RSV), and rhinovirus; fewer than 10 percent of the cases are caused by bacteria.

TYPES AND CAUSES OF BRONCHITIS IN WESTERN MEDICINE

Western medicine believes there are five types of bronchitis.

1. Acute bronchitis. This will last anywhere from several days to weeks, and will usually clear up on its own.
2. Viral bronchitis. This is triggered by a viral infection, such as the common cold.
3. Occupational bronchitis. People are exposed to lung irritants in the home or workplace and the treatment is usually to withdraw from the place.
4. Chronic bronchitis. Because the above symptoms last for longer than three months or recur frequently over a period of years, chronic bronchitis is not usually caused by infection, but is very of-

ten associated with chronic obstructive pulmonary disorder (COPD).

5. Asthmatic bronchitis has the same symptoms as bronchitis, but the underlying cause is asthma.

TREATMENT FOR BRONCHITIS IN WESTERN MEDICINE

By far the majority of bronchial cases are originally from viral infections, which means that most cases of bronchitis are short-term and require nothing more than symptomatic treatment. Since antibiotics do not cure a viral illness, overuse of antibiotics will make the bacteria that are accustomed to residing in the respiratory tract resistant to the antibiotics currently available. Many doctors prescribe antibiotics because they feel pressure from their patients. If they do not prescribe a certain antibiotic, they run the risk of their patients thinking they did nothing to help.

You can use acetaminophen, such as Tylenol, aspirin, or ibuprofen, to control the fever. Also you should drink as much fluid as possible in order to clear your body, dilute the virus, and make it dissipate in the body's fluid. A humidifier might help, and over-the-counter cough suppressants, such as Robitussin and Mucinex, might also assist in loosening the secretions.

Bronchodilator inhalers will help open airways and decrease the wheezing. If there is bacterial infection, antibiotics should be prescribed.

TREATMENT FOR BRONCHITIS IN TRADITIONAL CHINESE MEDICINE

Because there is no effective treatment for bronchitis from Western medicine, and the course of bronchitis usually takes about one week, traditional Chinese medicine (TCM) might play some important roles in healing or facilitating the recovery period. TCM believes that bronchitis is a lung disease, which results either from an attack of external disease factors, or from disorders of the lung itself.

For the invasion of outside disease factors, there are two types.

1. **Wind cold.** The main manifestations of this type are coughing, itching in the throat, and thick white sputum. The individual is easily susceptible to cold, with symptoms such as fever, headaches, nasal obstruction and discharge, and thirst, with thin white tongue coating and superficial pulse.
2. **Wind heat.** The main manifestations of this type are a choking cough with yellowish thick sputum, fever, headaches, sore throat, and thirst. Individuals experience an aversion to wind, they sweat, and they have a thin yellow coating on the tongue and a superficial, rapid pulse.

For the internal-organ injury of the lung, there are two types.

1. **Blockage of the lung by phlegm.** The main manifestation is coughing with profuse, thick white phlegm, loss of appetite, rolling pulse, stuffiness

and congestion of the chest, and white sticky tongue coating.

2. **Dryness of the lung with a deficiency of yin.** This is manifested by an afternoon fever, a dry cough without little or no sputum, dryness of the nose and throat, rapid pulse, red tongue with thick tongue coating, sore throat, and spitting, or even coughing up, blood.

Acupuncture for Bronchitis in Traditional Chinese Medicine

- For wind cold. You may choose acupuncture points, such as Lu 7 Lie Que, LI 4 He Gu, and UB13 Fei Shu (Lung Shu), with supplementary points Lu 11 Shao Shang for pain and swelling of the throat; and for fever and aversion to cold, Du 14 Da Zhui and SJ 5 Wai Guan.
- **For wind heat:** UB 13 Fei Shu, Lu 5 Qi Ze, Du 14 Da Zhui, LI 11 Qu Qi.

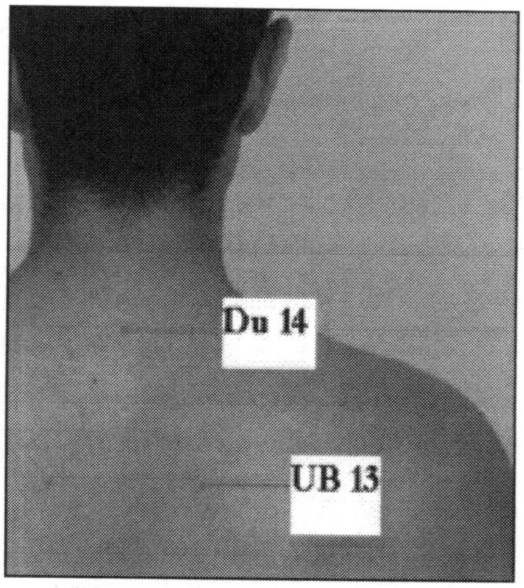

FIGURE 13.1

TABLE 13.1

POINTS	MERIDIAN NUMBER	CONDITIONS HELPED
Lie Que	Lu 7. See Figure 12.2	See Table 12.1
He Cu	LI 4. See Figure 12.3	See Table 12.1
Fei Shu	UB 13. See Figure 13.1	Cough, asthma, chest pain, spitting of blood, afternoon fever, night sweating
Shao Shang	Lu 11. See Figure 12.2	See Table 12.2
Da Zhui	Du 14. See Figure 12.1	See Table 12.2
VVai Guan	SJ 5. See Figure 12.3	See Table 12.2

Please refer to the accompanying Figures (illustrations) for the locations of the points. And please note that these illustrations are for information only and may not show all the exact locations of the acupuncture points.

TABLE 13.2

POINTS	MERIDIAN NUMBER	CONDITIONS HELPED
1 Fei Shu	UB 13. See Figure 13.1	See Fei Shu in Table 13.1
2 Qi Ze	Lu 5. See Figure 13.2	Cough, afternoon fever, asthma, sore throat, fullness in the chest, infantile convulsions, spasmodic pain of the elbow and arm
3 Da Zhui	Du 14. See Figure 12.1	See Table 12.2
4 Qu Qi	Li 11 See Figure 12.2	See Table 12.2

Please refer to the accompanying Figures (illustrations) for the locations of the points. And please note that these illustrations are for information only and may not show all the exact locations of the acupuncture points.

- For the internal lung injury with the blockage of the lung by phlegm, back-shu points and other lung points, such as UB 13 Fei Shu, Ren

12 Zhong Wan, Lu 5 Qi Ze, St 36 Zu San Li, and St 40 Feng Long are selected.

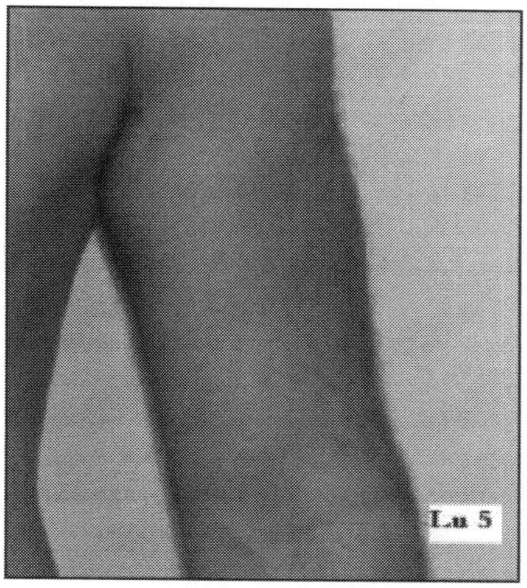

FIGURE 13.2

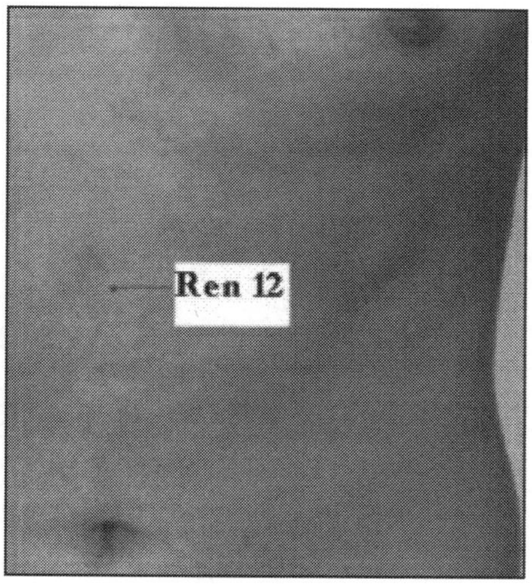

FIGURE 13.3

SUSAN'S TREATMENT

Susan was diagnosed as having wind cold, and after three days of treatment for this condition her symptoms disappeared and she returned to work.

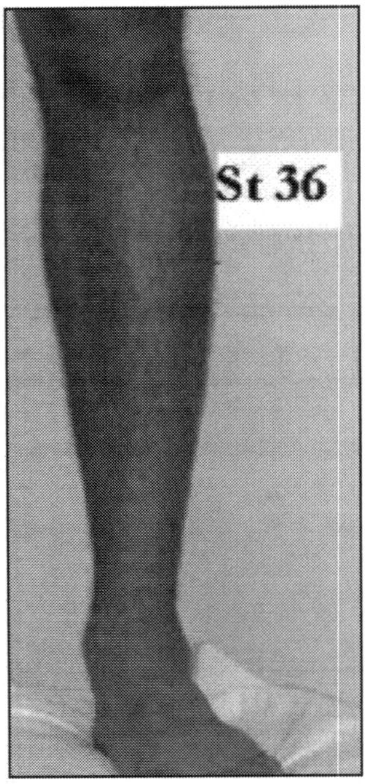

FIGURE 13.4

TABLE 13.3

POINTS	MERIDIAN NUMBER	CONDITIONS HELPED
1 Fei Shu	UB 13. See Figure 13.1	See Fei Shu in Table 13.1
2 Zhong Wan	Ren 12. See Figure 13.3	Stomach ache, abdominal distention, nausea, vomiting, acid reflex, diarrhea, dysentery, jaundice, indigestion, insomnia
3 Chi Ze	Lu 5. See Figure 13.2	See Chi Ze in Table 13.2
4 Zu San Li	St 36. See Figure 13.4	Gastric pain, vomiting, hiccups, abdominal distension, diarrhea, dysentery, constipation, aching of the knee joint and leg, edema, cough, asthma, emaciation indigestion, apoplexy, dizziness, insomnia

POINTS	MERIDIAN NUMBER	CONDITIONS HELPED
5 Feng Long	St 40. See Figure 13.4	Headaches, dizziness and vertigo, cough, asthma, excessive phlegm, pain in the chest, constipation, epilepsy, motor impairment, pain, swelling or paralysis of the lower extremities.

Please refer to the accompanying Figures (illustrations) for the locations of the points. And please note that these illustrations are for information only and may not show all the exact locations of the acupuncture points.

ACUPRESSURE TIPS TO USE AT HOME OR OFFICE

- The most important points are Fei Shu UB 13. Ask a friend or family member to press the points on both sides for 5 minutes each; alternately, press until you feel the flow of energy go through your lung.
- If you have a fever or feel very cold, press Da Zhui Du 14 for 10 minutes, then press Fei Shu UB 13. This will greatly improve your immune ability and quickly decrease your respiratory symptoms, such as coughing, or sneezing.

14

Asthma

YOUNG JIMMY HAS ASTHMA

Jimmy S. is a twelve-year-old boy who came to my office after a sudden onset of shortness of breath and tightness in the chest. In addition he said he had occasional pain and trouble sleeping, and listening to his lungs, I heard audible wheezing. He sometimes had coughs as well, and his mother reported he first developed these symptoms when he was two-years-old. The incidents happened mostly in cold weather, and sometimes when he ran or participated in sports. At these times he had difficulty in breathing, often coughed or wheezed, and all these symptoms together brought about a diagnosis of asthma. His doctor prescribed an inhaler and other medication, which made his asthma better for a while. However, although he used these asthma aids for a decade, he still had frequent attacks that made him miss classes, which bothered him, as he wanted to keep up with his schoolmates. His primary care physician could give him no further help, at which time he consulted me.

THE CAUSES OF ASTHMA

Asthma is an inflammation and constriction of the lungs and airways. The airways of a person with asthma are inflamed, to some degree, all the time. The more inflamed the airways are, the more sensitive they become.

People with asthma often have trouble breathing when they're in the presence of what are called triggers. Allergens, including dust, fur, mold, or perfumes, usually trigger asthma, as do cold air, irritants, such as smoke, physical activity, such as exercise, and respiratory infections, such as the common cold. Additionally, certain medications, such as aspirin and non-steroidal anti-inflammatory drugs (NSAIDs), can trigger asthma, as can allergic reactions to certain foods, gastroesophageal reflux disease (GERD), menstrual cycles, stress, and strong emotions.

When someone with asthma is exposed to these irritants and develops asthma symptoms, this means the flow of air is obstructed going in and out of the lungs because the lining of the airways becomes inflamed, which can produce extra mucus to block the irritants. This leads to inflammation that, in turn, causes the lining of the airways to constrict and block the repiratory tract.

The more inflammation there is, the more sensitive the airways become, and the more symptoms there are. The inflammation that makes it increasingly difficult for air to pass in and out of a person's lungs results in an increased difficulty in breathing and the onset of such asthma symptoms as coughing, shortness of breath, and wheezing. If the symptoms worsen, some people will get an infection, which will produce yellowish phlegm, and will, in turn, cause more severe symptoms.

Asthma is usually worse in the morning and late at night. In between asthmatic episodes, symptoms have been known to disappear or improve, but this does not mean the asthma has gone away, which is why Jimmy has had these symptoms for more than ten years.

THE FOUR TYPES OF ASTHMA IN WESTERN MEDICINE

1. Allergic asthma, caused by inflammation of the airway when exposed to allergens, such as dust, food, fur, mold, perfume, or smoking.
2. Exercise-induced asthma, which is triggered by vigorous activity.
3. Cough-variant asthma, which produces a chronic and persistent cough, sometimes called a habitual cough, without shortness of breath.
4. Occupational asthma, caused by exposure to stimulants, such as gas, oils, or certain chemicals in the workplace.

TREATMENTS IN WESTERN MEDICINE

In Western medicine, two types of medication treat asthma.

1. Bronchodilators, such as beta-agonist, albuterol, and salmeterol, and anticholinergics that block

the (contraction-inducing) neurotransmitter acetylcholine. These medications can dilate the respiratory tubes and open the lungs to air.

2. Corticosteroids. An inhaled corticosteroid is recommended for most people with asthma and is most effective for the respiratory tract, with minimal effect on the rest of the body at normal doses. If inhaled or given by injection, these are good for short-term relief to speed up the resolution of airway inflammation.

It is strongly recommended that people who have asthma carry their inhalers with them, in case of an emergency (this precaution sometimes plays a life or death role). For long-term treatment, however, Chinese medicine might be of more help.

TYPES OF ASTHMA IN TRADITIONAL CHINESE MEDICINE

Asthma is characterized by repeated attacks of shortness of breath with wheezing. It can be divided into two types: Excess and Deficiency.

Type 1—Excess

- **Wind cold.** This type of asthma attack is due to the invasion of a wind cold pathogen from the environment which impairs the smooth flow of the lung qi (energy), injures the skin and hair, and restricts or closes the respiratory tract, especially the bronchial tract. Since the lungs and the body's surface defense systems are weakened, the lung qi fails to disperse and descend, which leads to a cough.

- **Phlegm heat.** This type of asthma is due to the failure of the spleen to transform and transport, resulting in the production of phlegm from the accumulated dampness, and finally ending in the retention of phlegm. The phlegm causes the lungs to become hot and inflamed, impairing their ability to expel phlegm due to the stagnating condition of the lung energy (qi). And this is the cause of phlegm heat asthma.

Type 2—Deficiency

- **Lung deficiency.** A prolonged and protracted cough usually weakens and injures the lung energy, and straining an internal lung and respiratory muscle can also bring about deficiency of the lung energy. In either case, shortness of breath may occur.
- **Kidney deficiency.** Since the kidney is the energy resource of the human body, longstanding asthma, overwork, and other factors will affect the kidney function. Therefore, if there is a kidney deficiency, its energy cannot support lung functions, which will induce weakness of the kidney and make an asthma attack that much more severe.

ACUPUNCTURE TREATMENTS FOR TYPE 1 EXCESS ASTHMA

Wind Cold

For wind cold type, the principal is to keep away from exposure to cold and flu viruses, etc., as well as improve the lung's function and enrich the lung's energy. The acupuncture prescription for this is UB 13 Fei Shu, UB 12 Feng Men, Du 14 Da Zhui, Lu 7 Lie Que, LI 4 He Gu.

TABLE 14.1

POINTS	MERIDIAN NUMBER	CONDITIONS HELPED
1 Fei Shu	UB 13. See Figure 12.1	See Table 12.1; Figure 12.1
2 Feng Men	UB 12. See Figure 12.1	See Table 12.1; Figure 12.1
3 Da Zhui	Du 14. See Figure 12.1	See Table 12.2; Figure 12.1
4 Lie Que	Lu 7. See Figure 12.2	See Table 12.1; Figure 12.2
5 He Gu	LI 4. See Figure 12.3	See Table 12.1; Figure 12.3

Please refer to the accompanying Figures (illustrations) for the locations of the points. And please note that these illustrations are for information only and may not show all the exact locations of the acupuncture points.

ACUPRESSURE TIPS TO USE FOR TYPE 1 EXCESS ASTHMA AT HOME OR OFFICE Wind Cold

TABLE 14.2

POINTS	MERIDIAN NUMBER	CONDITIONS HELPED
1 Fei Shu	UB 13. See Figure 12.1	See Table 12.1, Figure 12.1
2 Ding Chuan	EX B 1. See Figure 14.1	Asthma, cough, neck rigidity, pain in the shoulder and back, German measles
3 Tian Tu	Ren 22. See Figure 14.2.	Asthma, cough, difficulty in swallowing, dry throat, goiter, hiccups, sore throat, sudden hoarseness of the voice
4 Qi Ze	Lu 5. See Figure 14.3	Afternoon fever, asthma, cough, fullness in the chest, infantile convulsions, sore throat, spasmodic pain of the elbow and arm
5 Feng Long	St 40. See Figure 14.4	Asthma, constipation, cough, dizziness and vertigo, epilepsy, excessive phlegm, general pain, headaches, motor impairment, muscular atrophy, pain in the chest, swelling or weakness of lower leg

Please refer to the accompanying Figures (illustrations) for the locations of the points. And please note that these illustrations are for information only and may not show all the exact locations of the acupuncture points.

- The most important points are UB 12, UB 13, and Du 14.

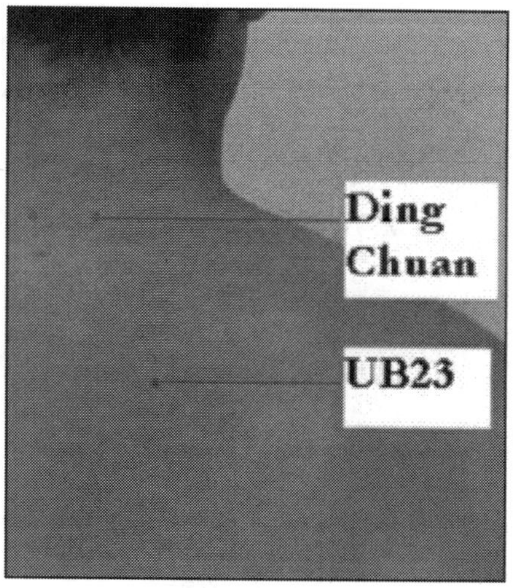

FIGURE 14.1

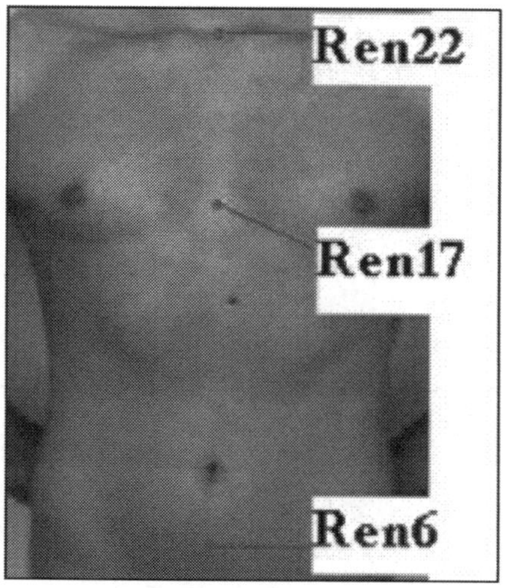

FIGURE 14.2

- Press UB 13 for 5 minutes with both your knuckles, then UB 12 for another 5 minutes. Alternate these about 3 times to help reduce the asthmatic symptoms and you might feel relief from this acupressure selftreatment.

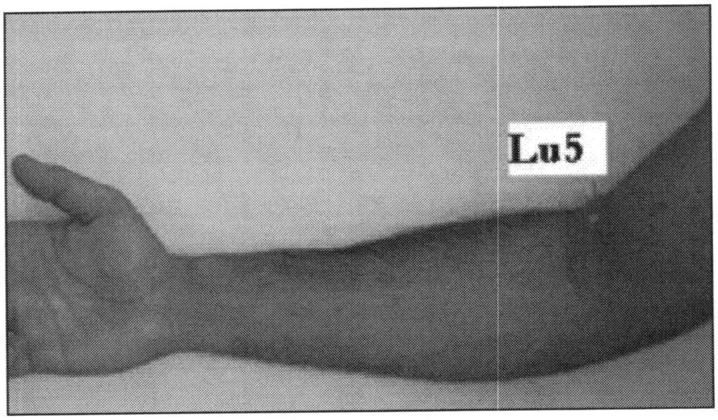

FIGURE 14.3

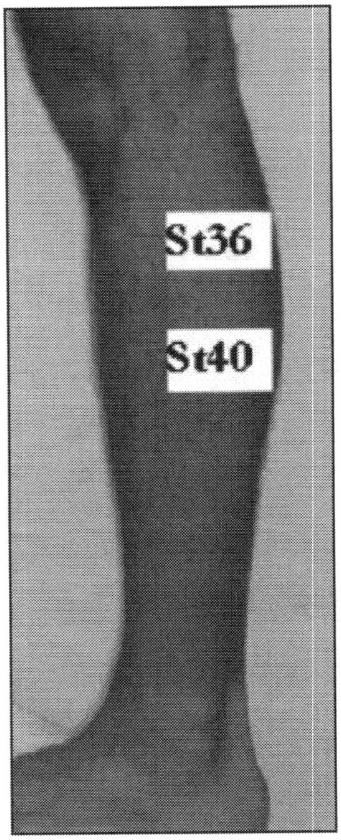

FIGURE 14.4

Phlegm Heat

- Press hard on bilateral EX B1 Ding Chuan for 5 minutes, then UB 13 Fei Shu for 5 minutes. Alternate for 2 sessions.

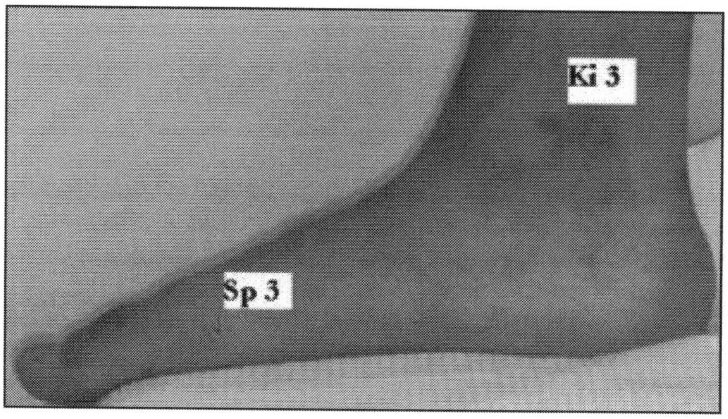

FIGURE 14.5

- Ren 22 Tian Tu may also help to decrease the asthma after pressing for about 5 minutes.

ACUPUNCTURE TREATMENTS FOR TYPE 2 DEFICIENCY ASTHMA

Lung Deficiency

The lung is the vital internal organ to regulate respiration. Lung energy deficiency leads to the easy entry of the pathogens, and causes asthma. The goal is to improve the lung energy and efficiency and decrease the chance of the body being attacked by exogenous pathogens.

TABLE 14.3

POINTS	MERIDIAN NUMBER	CONDITIONS HELPED
1 Fei Shu	UB 13. See Figure 12.1	See Table 12.1, Figure 12.1
2 Tai Yuan	Lu 9. See Figure 14.6	Cough, asthma, sore throat, palpitations, pain in the chest, wrist and arm
3 Zu San Li	St 36. See Figure 14.4	Gastric pain, vomiting hiccups, abdominal distension, diarrhea, dysentery, constipation, aching of the knee pint and leg, edema cough, asthma, emaciation due to general nutrition deficiency, indigestion, apoplexy, dizziness, insomnia, mania
4 Tai Bai	Sp 3. See Figure 14.5	Gastric pain, abdominal distension, constipation, dysentery, vomiting, diarrhea, sluggishness

Please refer to the accompanying Figures (illustrations) for the locations of the points. And please note that these illustrations are for information only and may not show all the exact locations of the acupuncture points.

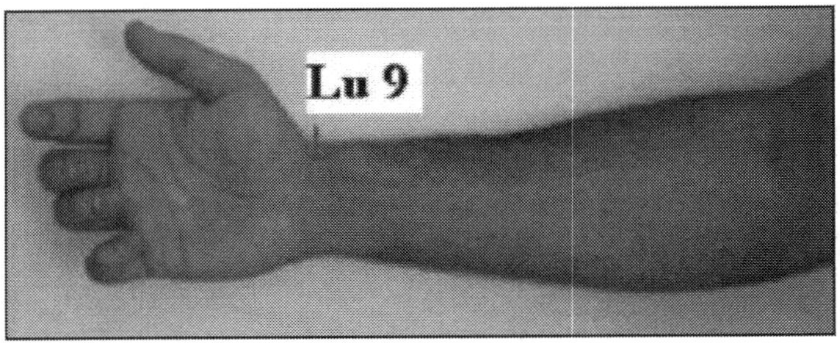

FIGURE 14.5

Kidney Deficiency

The kidney is the energy manufacturer of the entire human body. Any lessening of its function will cause a decrease of the immune function and energy flow of daily activity. For this reason it is necessary to strengthen the kidney.

- To strengthen the kidney, UB 13 Fei Shu, REN 17 Tan Zhong, K 3 Tai Xi and UB 23 Shen Shu, and Ren 6 Qi Hai are selected.

TABLE 14.4

POINTS	MERIDIAN NUMBER	CONDITIONS HELPED
1 Fei Shu	UB 13. See Figure 12.1	See Table 12.1, Figure 12.1
2 Tan Zhong	Ren 17. See Figure 14.2	Anorexia, distension and fullness in the chest and ribs, hiccups, nausea
3 Tai Xi	Ki 3. See Figure 14.5	Asthma, deafness, dizziness, impotence, insomnia, irregular menstruation, low back pain, nocturnal emissions, sore throat, thirst, tinnitus, toothache
4 Shen Shu	UB 23. See Figure 14.1	Asthma, blurred vision, deafness, diarrhea, dizziness, swelling, impotence, irregular menstruation, low back pain, nocturnal emissions, tinnitus, weakness of the knee

POINTS	MERIDIAN NUMBER	CONDITIONS HELPED
5 Qi Hai	Ren 6. See Figure 14.2	Abdominal pain, nocturnal emissions, impotence, hernia, edema, diarrhea, dysentery, uterine bleeding, irregular menstruation, postpartum hemorrhage, constipation, asthma

Please refer to the accompanying Figures (illustrations) for the locations of the points. And please note that these illustrations are for information only and may not show all the exact locations of the acupuncture points.

ACUPRESSURE TIPS TO USE FOR TYPE 2 DEFICIENCY ASTHMA AT HOME OR OFFICE

Lung Deficiency

- For long-term health care, always press St 36 and UB 13, even you do not have any illness; these two points will protect you from pathogens.
- Press Lu 9 and Sp 3 for an acute attack.

Kidney Deficiency

- UB 23 is the key point to press.
- UB 13 and Ren 17 will greatly help in strengthening the kidney function.
- NB: Acupressure the points with your thumb or knuckle, pressing with comfortable pressure on the points; count to 20, then change to another point.

You should work symmetric points at the same time.

ASTHMA THROUGH THE SEASONS IN TRADITIONAL CHINESE MEDICINE

Asthma attacks usually happen in the fall, winter, or spring, and only occasionally in the summer. In traditional Chinese medicine, summer is the most important season to reinforce the kidney and spleen yang energy. I insist that my patients have treatments during the summer. I use not only acupuncture, but also moxibustion (moxa) during the summer. One treatment in summer is probably the equivalent of four or five treatments in any other season. Utilizing the illustrated acupuncture points shown, it is possible to alleviate chronic asthmatic symptoms by strengthening the energy and improving the function of the spleen, as well as that of the stomach and kidneys. In this way, you can relieve, or even eradicate, future attacks.

JIMMY'S TREATMENT

Jimmy received a dozen treatments from me during the first summer he was my patient. The following school year his asthma was sufficiently under control to allow him to work very hard and do very well in his studies. Additionally, the summer treatments had helped him so much that he only needed to consult me for a few visits each summer after that.

15

Allergy and Sinusitis

DIAGNOSING ALLERGIES

Dan J was a sixteen-year-old boy who came to me complaining of itchy, pink eyes, difficulty breathing, headaches, and a runny nose which had exuded yellow and green sputum for two weeks. For more than five years, Dan had experienced these symptoms on and off—they got worse during the spring and autumn and better in the summer.

He was diagnosed with allergies that sometimes developed into sinusitis and was given Allegra, benadril and other antihistamine medications. In the beginning, this treatment helped, but after a week or two the medication stopped working. For more than a year, Dan was also given allergy shots with multiple antigens, but those didn't seem to work either.

His symptoms very often include severe sinusitis, headaches, poor sleep, and difficulty in concentration, and his physician often has to prescribe antibiotics to prevent an infection from developing further. Because of his mother's concern about his frequent use of antibiotics, he was brought to me, and he reported that he has all the symptoms listed above, plus a minor outbreak of hives on his face and body.

EXPLANATION OF ALLERGIES

Allergies are an abnormal reaction to an ordinary, harmless substance called an allergen. There are many different allergens, including dust, fur, mold, and pollen. When the allergens are absorbed into the body through breathing or skin contact, the immune system of a susceptible person will have a chain reaction, and the white blood cells will produce IgE antibodies. These antibodies attach themselves to mast cells, which will cause the release of histamine and other potent chemicals. This released histamine will cause a spasm of the smooth muscles in the respiratory tract, sinuses, skin, ears, and other parts of the body, which will lead to a runny nose, watery eyes, itching, and sneezing. If the sinus is infected with viruses and bacteria, sinusitis will occur and the person will develop a sinus headache and fever.

ALLERGIC REACTIONS IN WESTERN MEDICINE

There are five types of allergic reactions according to Western medicine.

1. Allergic rhinitis
2. Contact dermatitis
3. Eczema (atopic dermatitis)

4. Seasonal allergic rhinitis
5. Urtcaria (hives)

Symptoms can range from mild to severe and are usually treated with antihistamines, decongestants, cortisone products (which might produce long-term side effects), local chain modifiers, which will block the effects of inflammatory chemicals, and mast cell stabilizers.

ALLERGIC REACTIONS IN TRADITIONAL CHINESE MEDICINE (TCM)

Traditional Chinese medicine believes allergies and sinusitis are one disease, with two different manifestations and stages. In type 1, the first stage, the person's immune system is weakened. When the weather changes, such allergens as dust and mold increase and invade the body through the mouth, nose, and skin, causing symptoms in the lung and the liver. In type 2, the second stage, the allergies may induce further symptoms, such as a sinus infection, ear problems, or tinnitus. The person might have a low grade fever, a cough with yellow sputum, a headache, or insomnia.

Symptoms in the lung are shortness of breath and secretion from the sinuses because the nose is the opening for the lung. If there is an allergen invasion from outside, and the person's body is not strong enough to combat it—especially if the immune system is weakened—the weak immune system will make the lung symptoms worse. This is why different people can face the same allergen invasion and have different responses to it. Most people are not allergic to dust, mold, or the like. They have no problem with allergens. However, for those who do experience this condition, it is because their immune system is weakened and their body energy is low, especially in the lung.

The liver function corresponds to the eye, which is the outlet of the liver. If the liver function is low and weak, the eye symptoms, such as itchy, pink, and tearing eyes are more prominent.

TREATMENTS IN TRADITIONAL CHINESE MEDICINE

- Allergic sinusitis. Li 20 Ying Xiang is used, which corresponds to maxillary sinus, Li 11 Qu Qi, Li 4 He Gu, and GB 20 Feng Chi.
- Frontal sinusitis: add UB 2 Zan Zhu
- Ethmoid sinusitis: add SI 18 Quan Liao

ACUPRESSURE TIPS TO USE AT HOME OR OFFICE

Type 1 Allergy Sinusitis

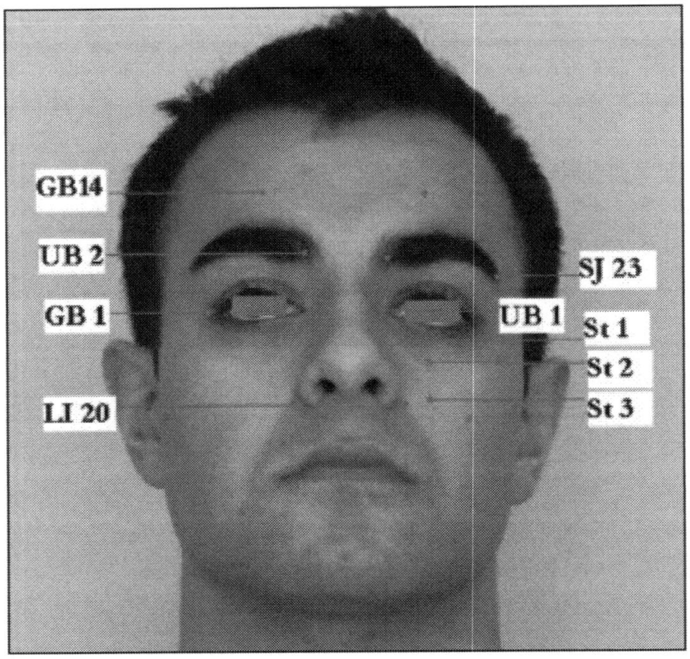

FIGURE 15.1. First Stage. The main symptoms for type 1 allergic sinusitis are sinusitis and headaches, so the acupuncture points for these symptoms are chosen.

TABLE 15.1

POINTS	MERIDIAN NUMBER	CONDITIONS HELPED
1 Ying Xiang	LI 20. See Figure 15.1	Nasal obstruction, insomia, facial paralysis, itching and swelling of the face
2 Ju Liao	St 3. See Figure 15.1	Facial paralysis, twitching of the eyelids, nosebleed, toothache, swelling of the lips and cheek

POINTS	MERIDIAN NUMBER	CONDITIONS HELPED
3 Qu Chi	LI 11. See Figure 12.2	Sore throat, toothache, eye redness and pain, scrofula (neck infection), hives, motor impairment of the upper extremities, abdominal pain, vomiting, diarrhea, diseases associated with fever
4 He Gu	LI 4. See Figure 12.2	Headaches, neck pain, pink, swelling, and painful eye, nosebleed, nasal obstruction, sweating, non–sweating, runny nose, toothache, deafness, swelling of the face, sore throat, facial paralysis, febrile (fever) diseases with abdominal pain, diarrhea, constipation, amenorrhea (no menstruation), delayed labor, infantile convulsions, pain, weakness, and motor impairment of the upper limbs.
5 Feng Chi	GB 20. See Figure 12.1	Headaches, dizziness, insomnia, neck pain and stiffness, blurred vision, glaucoma, pink and painful eyes, tinnitus, convulsions, epilepsy, infantile convulsions, febrile (fever) diseases, common cold, nasal obstruction, runny nose
6 Zan Zhu	UB 2. See Figure 1S.1	Headaches, blurred and poor vision, redness, swelling and pain of the eye, twitching of eyelids, glaucoma

POINTS	MERIDIAN NUMBER	CONDITIONS HELPED
7 Quan Liao	18. See Figure 15.2	Facial paralysis, twitching of eyelids, pain in the face, toothache, swelling of the cheek
8 Er Meng	SJ 21. See Figure 15.2	Tinnitus, deafness, toothache, stiffness of the lip.
9 Ting Gong	SI 19. See Figure 15.2	Deafness, tinnitus, motor impairment of the jaw, toothache
10 Ting Hui	GB 2. See Figure 15.2	Deafness, tinnitus, toothache, motor impairment of the jaw, mumps

Please refer to the accompanying Figures (illustrations) for the locations of the points. And please note that these illustrations are for information only and may not show all the exact locations of the acupuncture points.

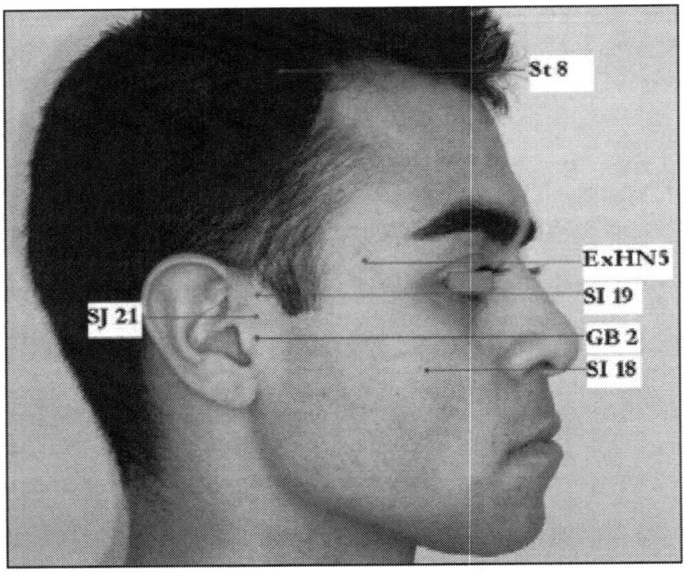

FIGURE 15.2. Second Stage. The main symptoms for type 2 allergy sinusitis are related to eye and ear problems, so the acupuncture points chosen are mainly for the eye and ear.

TABLE 15.2

POINTS	MERIDIAN NUMBER	CONDITIONS HELPED
1 Cheng Qi	St 1. See Figure 15.1	Redness, swelling, and pain of the eye, night blindness, twitching of eyelids, facial paralysis
2 Si Bai	St 2. See Figure 15.1	Redness, pain, and itching of the eye, facial paralysis, twitching of eye lids, pain in the face
3 Si Zu Kong	SJ 23. See Figure 15.1	Headaches, redness and pain of the eye, blurred vision, twitching of the eyelid, toothache, facial paralysis
4 Yang Bai	GB 14. See Figure 15.1	Headaches, eye pain, vertigo, twitching of the eyelids
5 Tong Zi Liao	GB 1. See Figure 15.1	Headaches, redness, and pain of the eyes, poor vision
6 Zan Zhu	UB 2. See Figure 1S.1	Headaches, blurred and poor vision, pain above the eyes, tearing, redness, swelling and pain of the eyes, twitching eyelids, glaucoma
7 ling Ming	UB 1. See Figure 1S.1	Redness, swelling and pain of the eye, night blindness, color blindness, blurred vision, nearsightedness
8 Tou Wei	St 8. See Figure 15.2	Headaches, blurred vision, tearing
9 Tai Yang	Ex–HN 5. See Figure 15.2	Headaches, eye diseases

Please refer to the accompanying Figures (illustrations) for the locations of the points. And please note that these illustrations are for information only and may not show all the exact locations of the acupuncture points.

- The key acupressure points are LI 20, UB 2, and GB 14. You will feel your sinus opening by pressing the above points on both sides for 5 minutes each, in 2–3 sessions.
- Irrigating your sinuses with normal saline or a Chinese herb solution, such as Xin Yi Hua, Cang Er Zi, might give you a significant improvement.

Type 2 Allergy Sinusitis

- For itching ear and tinnitus, SI 19, SJ 21, and GB 2 are the best choice. Press the above points for 3–5 minutes each, 2–3 sessions per day for 2 weeks and you will realize the beauty of the points.
- For tearing and itching eye, GB 1, UB 1, and St 1 are good choices.

NB: Acupressure the points with your thumb or knuckle, pressing with comfortable pressure on the points. You should work symmetric points at the same time.

DAN'S TREATMENT

Initially, Dan underwent my treatment for four visits. On his first visit, after about twenty minutes, his eyes were dry and his sinuses had stopped running, which made him happy and much more comfortable. With three more treatments, his symptoms were almost gone. After discussing the case with his mother, Dan came back for a total of ten more visits. His problem was mainly due to a weakened immune system with deficiency of both kidney and lung. He needed acupuncture to help him improve these systems and get rid off the effects of allergens on his body.

After his symptoms had subsided, Dan returned to my office for about twelve visits during the summer even though he did not have any symptoms. After these treatments, Dan's immune system was much strengthened, and he only needed to come to me for five or six visits at the start of the next allergy season. And recently his symptoms have improved so much that he no longer needs to consult me, even at the beginning of a new allergy season.

SEASONAL TREATMENTS

"Strengthen your yang during the summer, nourish your yin in the winter" is the wisdom of traditional Chinese medicine, which has guided TCM practitioners for more than two thousand years. It means that anyone who has allergies, asthma, or sinusitis should be treated during the summer to strengthen their yang—their immune system. The acupuncture points are UB 13 Fei Shu (lung), UB 15 Xin Shu (heart), UB 20 Pei Shu (spleen), and UB 23 Shen Shu (kidney). This is why I requested that Dan come to my office for twelve visits during the summer.

16

Smoking

SMOKING CESSATION

Steven W, a fifty-six-year-old man, is president and CEO of a large company. When he consulted me, it was due to his habit of smoking two packs of cigarettes a day for the past forty-five years. He had developed shortness of breath and heart palpitations and came to me hoping I could help him quit because he was afraid he might have lung cancer.

Steven is a heavy-set man who comes down hard on his feet and legs while walking, has yellowish facial skin, and smells of cigarettes, especially on his breath. He says he feels energetic, and by listening to his lungs, I ascertained there was no wheeze or cloud sound coming from the lung and his heartbeat was normal. In giving his history, Steven told me he had been in the army, and, after his tour of duty, had returned to the United States where he began working. Since he'd never gone to college, he knew he had to work extremely hard to beat his competitors. At 6AM, he roused both himself and his son (by telephone, as he worked in a different city) to go to work, and often he did not return home until 10PM. He worked like this seven days a week which, in the beginning, was doable. Recently, however, he had begun to feel he did not have the stamina to keep up this schedule and, fearful that he might die of smoking and working so hard, he came to me for help.

I impressed upon Steven the absolute necessity to stop smoking because, among other toxic effects, cigarettes contain the drug nicotine, which is as highly addictive as heroin, cocaine, or methamphetamines. Over time, the smoker becomes physically and emotionally addicted to nicotine and totally dependent on it. Many men think nicotine gives them the energy to support their lives, while many women believe cigarettes make, and keep, them thin. Studies have shown that smokers must deal with both physical and psychological dependence to be successful at quitting cigarettes and staying off them.

When a smoker inhales, nicotine is carried deep into the lungs where it is quickly absorbed into the bloodstream and then carried throughout the body. Nicotine affects many parts of the body, including the brain, the heart and blood vessels, the hormonal system, and the metabolism. It can be found in breast milk and even in the mucus secretions of smokers. Nicotine can freely enter the placenta during pregnancy and affect newborn infants.

Nicotine produces pleasant feelings that make the smoker want to smoke more and more, and after a while the smoker develops a tolerance to it, which results in increased smoking over time. The smoker reaches a certain nicotine level and then smokes to maintain this level.

PROBLEMS CAUSED BY SMOKING

Currently, all medical research indicates that many severe diseases are caused by smoking. These include bronchitis, emphysema, and even lung cancer, which makes many smokers try to cut back or quit altogether. However, as soon as a smoker does actually quit—for a few hours or a few days—withdrawal symptoms occur. These include anger, dizziness, depression, fatigue, feelings of frustration, headaches, impatience, increased appetite, irritability, restlessness, sleep disturbances, and trouble concentrating. All these symptoms can lead the smoker to start up again in order to boost nicotine levels in the blood back to the level where these symptoms do not exist.

In an effort to have Steven understand why he must quit, I made him aware of the following health issues.

- Although most everyone understands that smoking can cause lung cancer, there are many other cancers that can be introduced through smoking as well, including cancers of the mouth and vocal cords affecting the larynx, throat, and pharynx; leukemia, and cancers of the bladder, cervix, esophagus, kidneys, pancreas, and stomach.

- Lung disease can lead to pneumonia, chronic obstructive pulmonary disease (COPD), and chronic bronchitis.
- Smoking can also lead to blindness, blood-vessel diseases, heart attacks, and strokes.

DEFINITIONS OF SMOKING TYPES IN TRADITIONAL CHINESE MEDICINE

Chinese medicine believes that cigarette smoking falls into three major types.

- Type 1 is energy deficiency of the heart and lung, which includes bronchitis, coronary artery disease, emphysema, and insomnia. The main symptoms for this type are agitation, anxiety, asthmatic attacks, chest pain, coughs, insomnia and dreaming, shortness of breath, and sore throat.
- The second type is yin deficiency of the kidney and liver, which includes high blood pressure and insomnia. The main symptoms include dizziness, menstrual cramps, early ejaculation or night ejaculation, faintness, impotence, infertility, and tinnitus.
- The third type is weakness and deficiency of the spleen and stomach, which includes chronic gastritis and a peptic ulcer. The main symptoms include bloating, diarrhea, drowsiness, headaches,

heaviness of the body, poor appetite, and a stomach ache.

TREATMENTS IN TRADITIONAL CHINESE MEDICINE

A variety of acupuncture-related treatments have proven very helpful for people who are trying to quit smoking.

- Auricular acupuncture treatments—ear embedding needles. First, the most painful points on the ear are found, usually those corresponding to the heart and sympathetic system. I regularly use Sheng Meng, heart, lung, endocrine, and large intestine, and insert the needles at the auricular points. These needles stay in the ear for seven days, and I ask my patient to press the needles for 4–5 minutes per hour every day, which lessens the craving for the nicotine in a cigarette. He/she also presses the needles anytime there is the urge to smoke. It is possible to bathe or shower with the needles imbedded in the ear, but the person must be on the alert for any signs of inflammation or infection.
- Laser treatment. Laser needles can also be used on the auricular acupuncture point, aiming directly at the ear for usually 2–3 minutes. For each treatment, four points are used for 15 minutes each time, with the total treatment time about

25–30 minutes. This is done 3 times a week for 4–8 weeks.

- Auricular acupuncture point injections. Sodium chloride (0.5 percent) can be injected each day in one or two points, always changing the points after each injection. Endocrine, Sheng Meng, Stomach, Liver, and Lung points are often used.
- Electrical stimulation for the ear. I usually select Sheng Meng, Lung, and Endocrine, and use a 1-inch needle in both ears. I do six points, then employ electrical stimulation for about 30 minutes and continue this treatment every other day for a total of four weeks.
- Body acupuncture. Emotional burdens, such as anxiety, depression, poor sleep, and stress, can force many people to smoke; therefore, body acupuncture can help to reduce emotional problems.

Type 1 Treatments—Energy Deficiency of the Heart and Lung

For energy deficiency of the heart and lung, auricular points are Heart, (Sympathetic), Sheng Meng; body points are Lu1 Zhong Fu, Renl6 Ju Que, Pc 6 Nei Guan, UB13 Fei Shu, UB15 Xin Shu, Sp 6 San Yin Jiao, and Lu5 Chi Zhe.

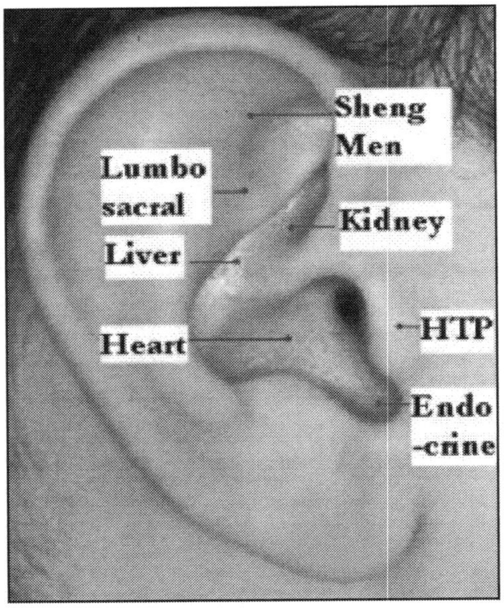

FIGURE 16.1

TABLE 16.1

POINTS	MERIDIAN NUMBER	CONDITIONS HELPED
1 Heart	Auricular. See Figure 16.1	Generalized heart disease
2 Sympathetic	Auricular. See Figure 16.1	Emotional problems, creating calm
3 Sheng Men	Auricular. See Figure 16.1	Emotional problems, creating calm
4 Hunger/Thirst Point	Auricular (HTP). See Figure 16.1	Supressing a craving for food, drugs, and alcohol
5 Zhong Fu	Lu I. See Figure 16.2	Asthma, cough, fullness of the chest, pain in the back, chest, and shoulder
6 Ju Que	Ren 14. See Figure 16.2.	Acid regurgitation, difficulty in swallowing, epilepsy, mental disorders, nausea, pain in the cardiac region and chest, palpitations, vomiting

POINTS	MERIDIAN NUMBER	CONDITIONS HELPED
7 Nei Guan	PC 6. See Figure 16.7	Cardiac pain, epilepsy, hiccups, insomnia, irritability, mental disorders, nausea, palpitations, stomach ache, stuffy chest, vomiting, malaria, contracture and pain in the elbow and arm.
8 Fei Shu	UB 13. See Figure 13.1	See Table 13.1, Figure 13.1
9 Xin Shu	UB IS. See Figure 16.3	Loss of memory, palpitations, cough, spitting up blood, nocturnal emissions, night sweats, epilepsy
10 San Yin Jiao	Sp 6. See Figure 16.6	Abdominal pain, diarrhea, uterine bleeding, prolapse of the uterus, delayed labor, nocturnal emissions, impotence, swelling, hernia, pain in the external genitalia, muscular atrophy, motor impairment, paralysis and pain in the lower extremities, headaches, dizziness and vertigo, insomnia
11 Qi Zhe	Lu 5. See Figure 13.2	See Table 13.2; Figure 13.2

Please refer to the accompanying Figures (illustrations) for the locations of the points. And please note that these illustrations are for information only and may not show all the exact locations of the acupuncture points.

Type 2 Treatments—Yin Deficiency of the Kidney and Liver

For yin deficiency of the kidney and liver, auricular (ear) points are the Kidney, Liver, Sheng

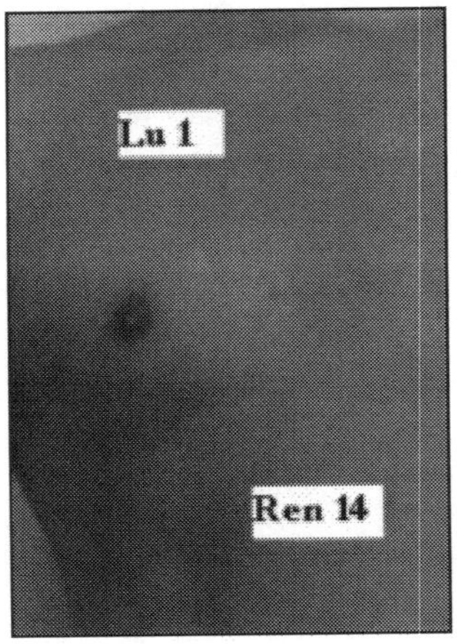

FIGURE 16.2

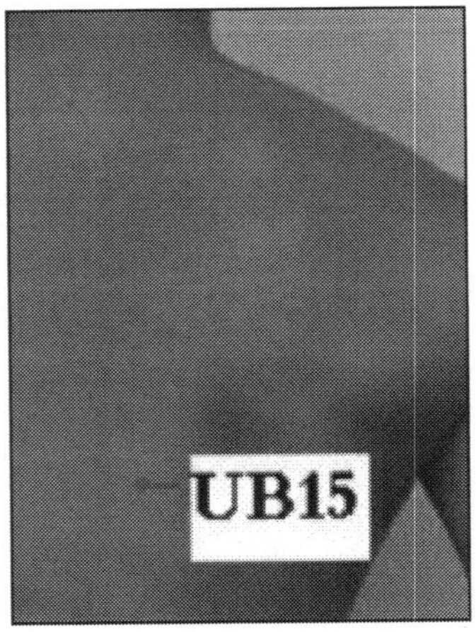

FIGURE 16.3

Meng, and Endocrine; body points are UBl Jing Meng, Liv2 Xing Jian, Kid3 Tai Xi, UB18 Gan Shu, Du20 Bai Hui, and Kid5 Shui Quan.

In my experience, the first two weeks of trying to stop smoking are the most crucial time because that is when the nicotine withdrawal syndrome is the most severe. The person withdrawing can be agitated, depressed, anxious, and have insomnia, and any of these can cause a return to smoking.

If I treat a patient with ear acupuncture, she/he can constantly press the needles embedded in the ear, which will decrease the craving for a cigarette and reinforce the psychological support. If the smoker knows all the consequences of smoking and wants to quit, this can usually be accomplished with acupuncture. Most succeed with the right attitude about the consequences of continuing to smoke.

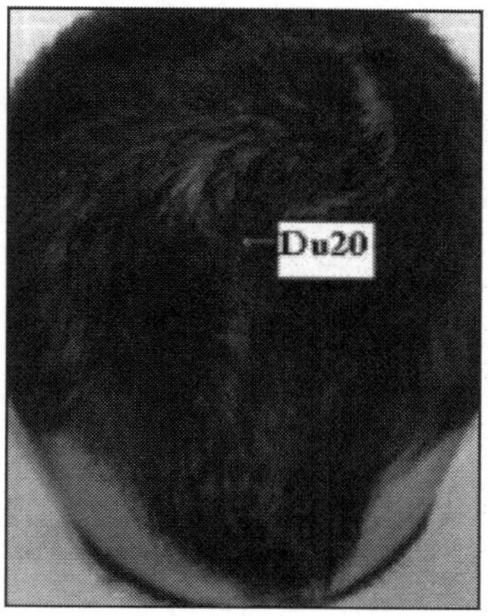

FIGURE 16.4

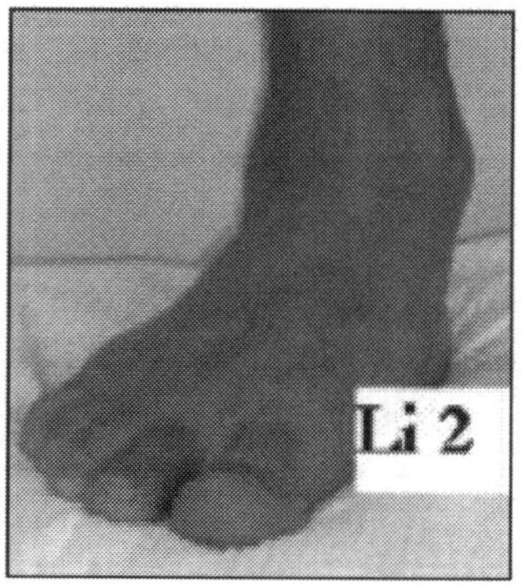

FIGURE 16.5

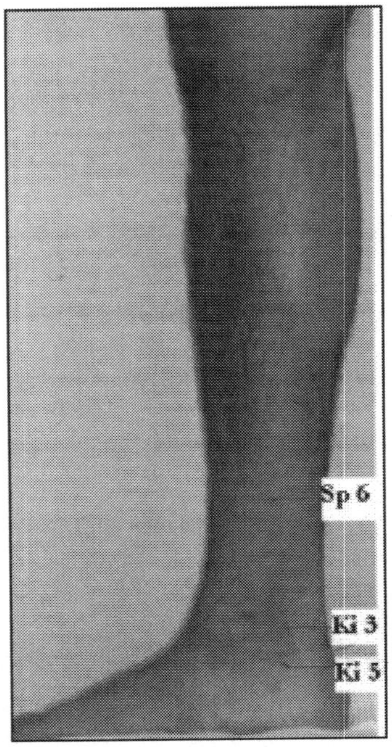

FIGURE 16.6

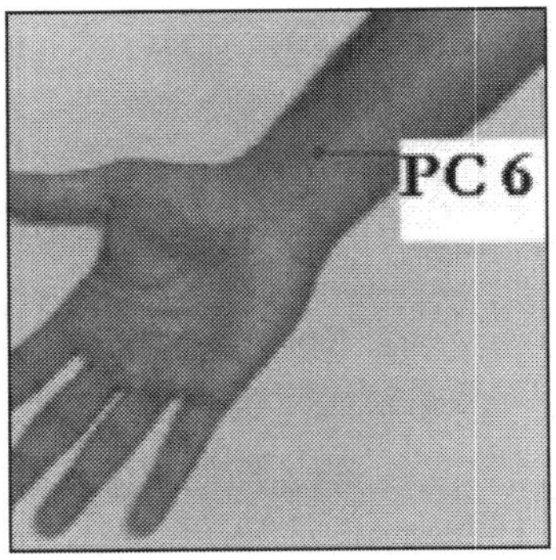

FIGURE 16.7

TABLE 16.2

POINTS	MERIDIAN NUMBER	CONDITIONS HELPED
I Liver	Auricular. See Figure 16.1	Generalized liver disease
2 Kidney	Auricular. See Figure 16.1	Generalized kidney disease
3 Sheng Meng	Auricular. See Figure 16.1	Emotional problems, creating calm

POINTS	MERIDIAN NUMBER	CONDITIONS HELPED
4 Endocrine	Auricular. See Figure 16.1	Endocrine disorders
5 Hungers/Thirst Point	Auricular. See Figure 16.1	Supressing a craving for food, drugs, and alcohol
6 Xing Jian	Liver 2. See Figure 16.5	Abdominal problems, congestion, convulsions, dizziness and vertigo, epilepsy, eye pain and swelling, headaches, hernia, insomnia, painful urination, urinary retention
7 Tai Xi	Kidney 3. See Figure 16.3	Asthma, deafness, dizziness, irregular menstruation, sore throat, spitting up blood, thirst, tinnitus, toothache, insomnia, nocturnal emissions, impotence, low back pain
8 Sheng Shu	UB 23. See Figure 14.1	See Table 14.4, Figure 14.1
9 Bai Hui	Du 20. See Figure 16.4	Headaches, vertigo, tinnitus, nasal obstruction, coma, mental disorders, prolapse of the rectum and uterus
10 Shui Quan	Kidney 5. See Figure 16.6	Irregular menstruation, prolapse of uterus, blurred vision

Please refer to the accompanying Figures (illustrations) for the locations of the points. And please note that these illustrations are for information only and may not show all the exact locations of the acupuncture points.

STEVEN'S TREATMENT

Steven was treated with both ear (auricular) and body acupuncture. He had three treatments a week for eight weeks. After the first week, he reduced his intake to one pack of cigarettes a day, and the second week, he stopped smoking. After a total time of eight weeks, he was completely off cigarettes.

TIPS TO STOP SMOKING

- Be determined and stick to the program. The first two weeks are the most difficult time. If you can stick to it, you will win the war.
- Think about your future and your family's future. You do not want to set up a wrong role model for your children and family members nor do you want to make them ill with secondhand smoke.

17

Drug Abuse

DRUG ABUSER

Peter W. is a fifty-three-year-old man who has been extremely successful in business. During his career, he built up a huge company which he sold for 20 million dollars in 2000. Afterward, he felt depressed and realized he had nothing to do, which made him sluggish and without motivation, as he had no goal to pursue. He started using drugs, including heroin, and it soon became a daily habit. When he was no longer able to procure drugs easily in the United States, he turned to the Internet and started ordering drugs by email, which were sent to him from Africa. Though he had no real idea what he was using, he continued with his habit, which made him feel empty, depressed, anxious and restless, and gave him insomnia, all of which caused a poor relationship with his wife and family. On some occasions he used so heavily he was unable to rise from his bed for a couple of days, on other occasions his family had to rush him to the emergency room. He felt occasional euphoria, followed by deep depression and cloudy mental functioning.

He knew this was no way to live, so he tried to find work that would engross him. For example, he took a volunteer job and helped the company build $100.00 laptop computers for distribution in third world countries to help the young people there. In spite of this worthwhile work, he still felt empty. He took another job as a V.P., with a seat on the Board of Directors, in one of the biggest computer companies. He worked very hard at this new job, but as soon as he stopped working or had leisure time, he found himself reverting to drug use. Finally, he came to me for help, saying he wanted to quit drugs altogether.

Heroin is a highly addictive, illegal drug, the most abused and most rapid-acting of the opioids. It is processed from morphine and a naturally occurring substance extracted from the seeds of certain varieties of poppy plants. It usually appears as white or brown powder, and is sometimes mixed with sugar and other substances to cut its strength.

Heroin has both long- and short-term effects. The short-term effects include poor respiration, clouded mental functions, depression, nausea, spontaneous abortion, and vomiting. It is used medicinally for the suppression of pain, though under controlled conditions. In addition, heroin can cause temporary feelings of euphoria. Long-term effects include addiction and infectious diseases, such as abscesses, arthritis, bacterial infections, collapsed veins, hepatitis B and C, HIV/AIDS, and pneumatic problems.

TREATMENTS IN WESTERN MEDICINE

In Western medicine there are many types of detoxification programs. Methadone, the most popular, is a synthetic opioid that blocks the effects of the heroin and eliminates withdrawal symptoms. This method has a proven record of success for heroin addicts.

The drug buprenorphine is a pharmaceutical approach to behavioral therapy. It offers less risk than methadone and can be prescribed in the doctor's office. Bupherorphine and Suboxone make up a combination drug product that is formulated to minimize abuse.

TREATMENTS IN TRADITIONAL CHINESE MEDICINE

Chinese medicine and acupuncture have a long history of treating drug abuse. The two types of treatments are:

- Auricular (ear) acupuncture;
- Body acupuncture.

The main functions of acupuncture treatments for drugs are to decrease the withdrawal symptoms and improve the person's brain function and depression. There are many studies supporting these treatments, and the most widely known study found that acupuncture can directly increase the level of the endogenous endorphins, which can make a person feel calm, relaxed, and cheerful. Acupuncture can also directly stimulate the central nervous system to lessen the craving for drugs and make a person feel less depressed.

Auricular Acupuncture

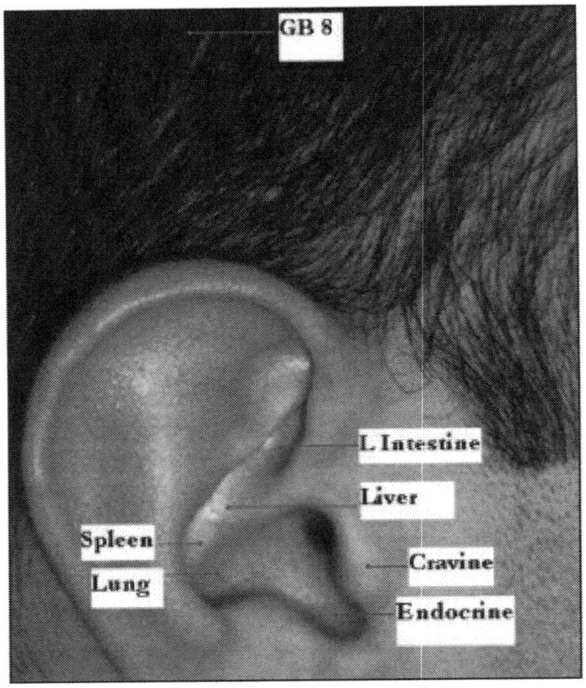

FIGURE 17.1

For auricular acupuncture, I use the Lung, Endocrine, Liver, Spleen, and Large Intestine points corresponding to these organs. The lung has an opening through the nose and when people abuse heroin, the Lung point will protect the lung function and strengthen the immune system. The Endocrine points increase endorphin secretion and increase the immune system's function of protecting the entire body. Liver and Spleen points improve circulation and also improve the taste in the mouth because the spleen and stomach have openings in the mouth and Large Intestine points. The intestine and the lung have a direct meridian connection, so if the function of the large intestine is improved, this will, in turn, directly improve the lung function.

TABLE 17.1

POINTS	MERIDIAN NUMBER	CONDITIONS HELPED
1 Lung	Auricular. See Figures 16.1, 17.1	Generalized lung diseases
2 Endocrine	Auricular. See Figures 16.1, 17.1	Generalized endocrine disorders
3 Liver	Auricular. See Figures 16.1, 17.1	Generalized liver diseases
4 Spleen	Auricular. See Figures 16.1, 17.1	Generalized spleen diseases
5 Large Intestine	Auricular. See Figures 16.1, 17.1	Generalized large intestine diseases
6 Hunger/Thirst Craving Points	Auricular. See Figures 16.1, 17.1	Supressing a craving for food, drugs, and alcohol

Please refer to the accompanying Figures (illustrations) for the locations of the points. And please note that these illustrations are for information only and may not show all the exact locations of the acupuncture points.

Body Acupuncture

For the body acupuncture points, the most important ones are on the head. I use DU 20 Bai Hui plus Extn 1 Shi Sheng Chong, total five points, which can directly stimulate the central nervous system when I add electrical stimulation to the needles. They send current directly to the cortex of the brain, which greatly decreases depression and improves a person's mood. GB 8 Shuai Gu, on the head 1.5 inches above the tip of the auricular, is directly connected to the sensory cortex, which will improve the body's sensation and make it dislike the taste of heroin. LI 4 He Gu is a point that can largely increase endorphin secretion and LI 11 Qu Chi will give a better functioning effect. PC 6 Nei Guan is a point of the pericardium meridian that also helps improve mental functions. Lu 7 Lie Que is the point from the lung meridian that protects the lung from attacks of heroin and improves the immune function of the lung.

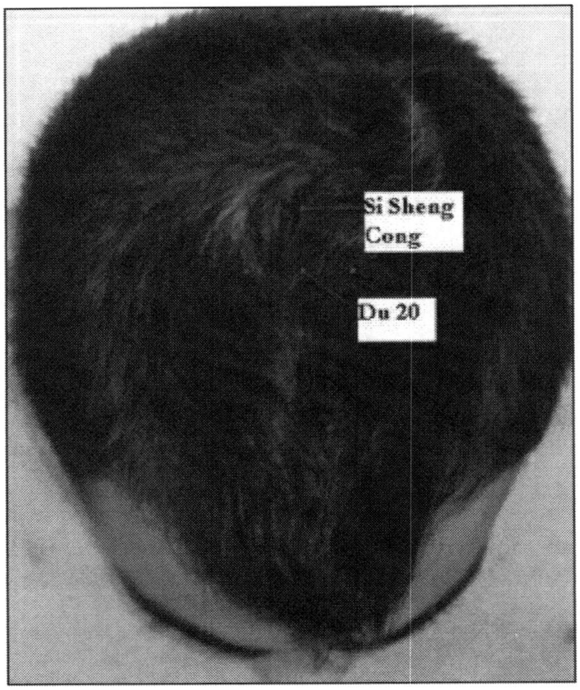

FIGURE 17.2

TABLE 17.2

POINTS	MERIDIAN NUMBER	CONDITIONS HELPED
1 Bai Hui	Du 20. See Figure 16.4	See Table 16.2, Figure 16.4
2 Si Sheng Cong	Ex–HN 1. See Figure 17.2	Epilepsy, headaches, insomnia, poor memory, vertigo
3 Shuai Gu	GB 8. See Figure 17.1	Infantile convulsions, migraine, vertigo, vomiting
4 He Gu	LI 4. See Figure 12.2	See Table 12.1
5 Qu Qi	LI 11. See Figure 12.2	See Table 12.1
6 Nei Guang	PC 6. See Figure 16.7	See Table 16.1, Figure 16.7
7 Lie Que	Lu 7. See Figure 12.2	See Table 12.1

Please refer to the accompanying Figures (illustrations) for the locations of the points. And please note that these illustrations are for information only and may not show all the exact locations of the acupuncture points.

PETER'S TREATMENTS

After two weeks of treatment, Peter's withdrawal symptoms started to decrease and he had more energy. I continued the acupuncture treatments three to four times a week for eight weeks, while also discussing the short and long-term effects of heroin use and what organs would be affected and harmed by continued use. At that point, he still felt cravings for heroin, and had some physical weakness, with muscle spasms in his arms and legs. He also experienced restlessness and agitation, often accompanied by insomnia.

In spite of the withdrawal symptoms Peter still experienced, he said the treatments made him feel much better. He was happy to treat his addiction in this fashion rather than go into a methadone program, which would have made his drug use generally known. By coming to me, he could be treated for his addiction in private.

In our ongoing discussions, I advised Peter to make lifestyle adjustments, and encouraged him to resume the volunteer work he had been doing. He traveled to Africa and Asia to actually meet the people using the inexpensive computers he had helped to build, and see for himself how these little electronic machines had improved their lifestyles. This experience touched him a great deal, and after about three months of treatment he stopped using heroin entirely and is now completely clean. His insomnia, depression, anxiety, and other symptoms are much improved and he is again leading a normal life.

18

Gastritis

JEFFREY'S GASTRITIS SYMPTOMS

Jeffrey, a forty-five-year-old-man, was brought into my office by his wife who was frankly at her wit's end. She had called me earlier to say her husband had awakened that morning with a sudden onset of burning, gnawing pain in his stomach that he thought was probably due to hunger. But, after drinking some milk and eating two pieces of bread, the pain got worse and he became nauseous and vomited. He was bloated and the pain was so strong he was not able to sit down, so he asked his wife to take him to the emergency room. She called me before doing so, and I told her to bring him right in.

While taking his case history, he told me of the same pains and symptoms as his wife, and he also told me he'd had a normal bowel movement that morning. I was puzzled by his condition, so outside his hearing I consulted further with his wife.

She told me that three days before their visit to me, she had called Jeffrey at his office, telling him to come home immediately. The IRS had arrived with orders to seal the house, due to ten years of unpaid income taxes. They had sent Jeffrey a letter, to which he had not responded, warning about the consequences of not paying his back taxes. The family was given two days to clean out and vacate the house. To compound this disaster, Jeffrey's partners were forced to sever the partnership, owing to his not filing taxes for a decade; his reputation had suffered to such a degree they could no longer remain in business with him. So, within three days, Jeffrey had lost his job, his income, and his house, and was under a tremendous amount of stress. His stress and nausea that morning had caused so much pain that he was crying and screaming, which is why his wife called me.

I returned to Jeffrey and asked if he had any other complaints besides the bad stomach with all its ramifications. He told me he was terribly depressed and stressed out, and he had no idea where to turn next. He was very agitated, so I had to ask him to calm down and let me examine him.

I first checked his stomach, which was soft, but there seemed no increase in bowel sound and no rebound pain. Owing to the events of the previous few days, however, Jeffrey may have experienced stress that was so overwhelming he may not have been able to tolerate it, and that caused him to develop acute stress gastritis, a condition that decreases blood flow to the stomach, impairing the lining of the stomach wall and hampering its ability to protect or renew itself. This can, in turn, lead to erosive gastritis. Although it's not clear what the exact mechanism is that will allow acute stress from the outside to cause decreased blood flow to the stomach's wall, in Jeffrey's case, stress was probably the root cause.

THE CAUSES OF GASTRITIS

- Infectious bacteria, viruses, or fungi are leading causes. It is well known that helicobacter pylori bacteria are the most common cause of gastritis and peptic ulcer. H. pylori bacteria can survive in a highly acidic environment and when they invade the stomach wall, they cause gastric acid to erode the stomach wall and this causes gastritis and a peptic ulcer. Other viruses can also develop in the gastric wall and impair the immune system in those who have AIDS or cancer, or those using immunosuppressive drugs.
- Erosive gastritis involves post-inflammation pathological changes in the stomach wall, and the wearing away of the stomach lining in anyone taking such drugs as aspirin and other non-steroidal anti-inflammatory drugs (NSAIDs). In some cases, even baby aspirin taken daily can injure the stomach lining.
- Acute stress gastritis, a form of erosive gastritis, is caused by the sudden onset of emotional damage. The injury might not even be to the stomach; it could be caused by severe stress and depression, extensive skin burns, or injuries involving major illnesses that cause bleeding.

- Radiation gastritis can occur if radiation is delivered to the lower left side of the chest.
- Atrophic gastritis. This is either caused by a chronic infection of H. pylori, or it can result from the surgical removal of any part of the stomach, due to the auto-antibody (the antibody produced by your own body), attacking the lining of the stomach wall.
- Other types of gastritis include eosinophilic gastritis, lymphocytic gastritis, and Menière's disease gastritis.

TREATMENT OF GASTRITIS IN WESTERN MEDICINE

From Western medicine's point of view, there are three major routes to treating gastritis:

- Antacids. Over-the-counter treatments, such as Maalox or Mylanta in liquid or tablet form, are the common treatment for mild gastritis. Antacids neutralize stomach acid and can provide fast pain relief.
- Acid blockers, such as famotidine, nizatidine, Pepcid, rantidine, Tagamet, and Zantac, help reduce the amount of acid the stomach produces. There are also pump blocks, such as Aciphex, Nexium, Prevacid, and Prilosec, which can inhibit the proton pump and reduce acid.
- Treating H. pylori most often involves a combination of two antibiotics and one proton-pump in-

hibitor. The antibiotics help destroy the bacteria and the proton-pump inhibitor relieves pain and nausea while healing inflammation and may also increase the effectiveness of the antibiotic.

TREATMENT OF GASTRITIS IN TRADITIONAL CHINESE MEDICINE

From the Chinese medicine point of view, a stomach ache manifests itself in repetitive and recurrent pain accompanied by acid reflux, nausea, passing gas, and vomiting.

Causes of Stomach Pain

Chinese medicine believes there are four causes of stomach pain.

- **Cold.** The coldness, sometimes caused by drinking too many cold liquids, directly attacks the stomach. This combination of internal cold and external cold will block the stomach qi (energy) and decrease the stomach movement, therefore to lead to a stomach ache.
- **Improper diet.** Overeating, starvation, or any irregular diet can cause stomach pain, resulting in contractions that make the stomach energy slow down, along with making the person feel fullness and bloating.
- **Emotional stress.** In today's world, almost everyone is under some stress. Some people cannot handle this stress, and when it becomes overwhelm-

ing, it will attack the stomach functions. The liver is the key regulator for emotion and energy (qi). If the liver's functions are blocked because of anxiety, depression, emotional stress, or panic, the liver cannot regulate the stomach energy or improve the stomach movement, and this results in stomach pain.

- **Excessive work** and fatigue can lead to stomach injury, which, in turn, can decrease the yin in the stomach and cause pain. The person usually feels hungry, and has, as well, a full, bloating sensation, a bad smell in the mouth, and a yellow, thick coating on the tongue.

Treating the Pain of Acute Illness

In Chinese medicine, the principal idea is to treat the pain for acute illness, and treat the cause of chronic illness.

- **Acute pain.** Its major manifestation is a sudden onset, acute stomach ache. It frequently occurs, causing distention of the stomach that makes it extremely tender to the touch. In this case, the principal of acupuncture is to decrease the pain and improve the energy flow. The points of acupuncture are Ren 12 Zhong Wan, St 36 Zusanli. These points warm the middle stomach and regulate the smooth muscle of the stomach rhythm, improving the qi (energy) of the stomach. PC 6 Nei Guan and Sp 4 Gong Sun can decrease nausea and improve the stomach, and even the large intestine, movement. Sp 9 Ying Ling Quan is the point which will help to decrease acid reflux.

TABLE 18.1

POINTS	MERIDIAN NUMBER	CONDITIONS HELPED
1 Zhong Wan	Ren 12. See Figure 13.3	See Table 13.3
2 Zhu San Li	St 36. See Figure 13.4	See Table 13.3
3 Nei Guang	PC 6. See Figure 18.1	Chest bloating, chest pain, epilepsy, hiccups, insomnia, irritability, mental disorders, nausea, pain of the elbow and arm palpitations, stomach pain, vomiting
4 Gong Sun	Sp 4. See Figure 18.2	Abdominal pain, diarrhea, dysentery, gastric pain, vomiting
5 Ying Ling Quan	Sp 9. See Figure 18.2	Abdominal pain, diarrhea, dysentery, swelling, incontinence, jaundice, pain in the external genitalia, pain in the knee
6 Shen Shu	UB 23. See Figure 18.3	See Table 14.4
7 Pi Shu	UB 20. See Figure 18.3	Jaundice, vomiting, diarrhea, dysentery, bloody stools, profuse menstruation, swelling, anorexia, back pain
8 Tai Chong	Li 3. See Figure 18.2	Headaches, dizziness and vertigo, insomnia, congestion, swelling and pain of the eye, depression, uterine bleeding retention of urine, epilepsy
9 Zhang Meng	Li 13. See Figure 18.4	Diarrhea, indigestion, vomiting

POINTS	MERIDIAN NUMBER	CONDITIONS HELPED
10 Tian Shu	St 25. See Figure 18.4	Abdominal pain and distention, pain around the navel, constipation, diarrhea, dysentery, irregular menstruation, swelling
I 1 Nei Ting	St 44. See Figure 18.2	Toothache, pain in the face, sore throat, nosebleed, gastric pain, acid regurgitation, bloating, diarrhea, dysentery, constipation, swelling and pain of the foot

Please refer to the accompanying Figures (illustrations) for the locations of the points. And please note that these illustrations are for information only and may not show all the exact locations of the acupuncture points.

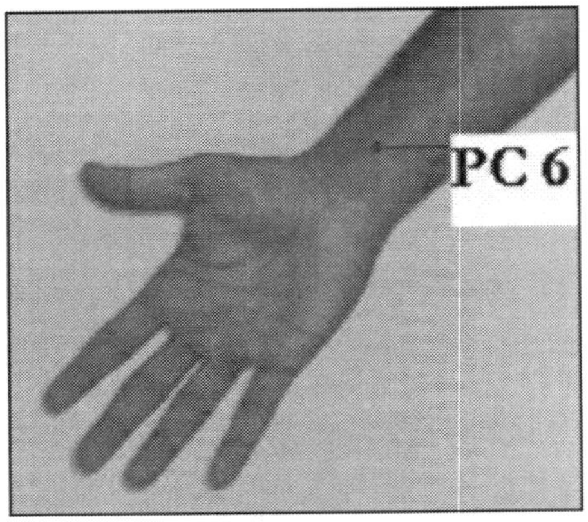

FIGURE 18.1

Treating the Chronic Illnesses

- **Chronic illness: Spleen and stomach deficiency.** The major symptoms here are diarrhea, fatigue, a mild though prolonged stomach ache, and stomach bloating. The treatment is to warm the stomach and improve the yin. The acupuncture points are Ren12 Zhong Wan, St 36 Zu San Li, PC 6 Nei Guan, UB 23 Sheng Shu and UB 20 Pi Shu. Sheng Shu and Pi Shu can help improve the yang of the stomach and kidney, improve the secretion of blood, and increase the energy flow in the stomach and the spleen, stimulating the function of the spleen and stomach.

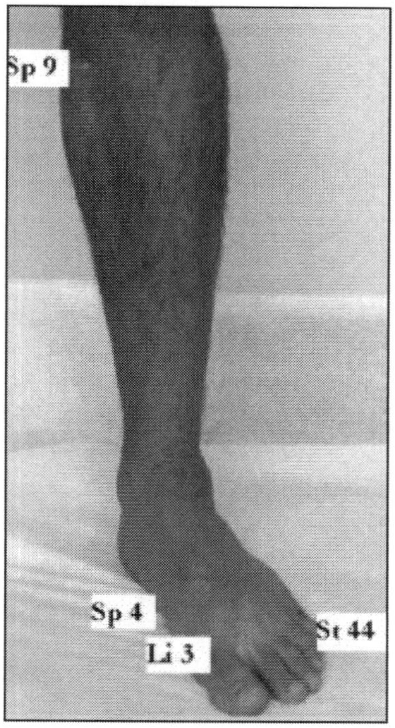

FIGURE 18.2

- **Chronic illness: Excessive liver energy attacking the stomach.** This is the type of Jeffrey's symptoms. The main manifestation is pain in the stomach and abdomen, accompanied by symptoms of excessive liver energy, such as dry mouth, bitter mouth, headaches, and high blood pressure, with the stomach

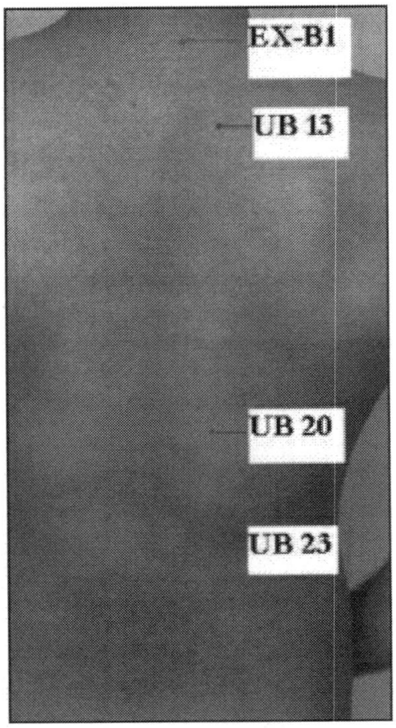

FIGURE 18.3

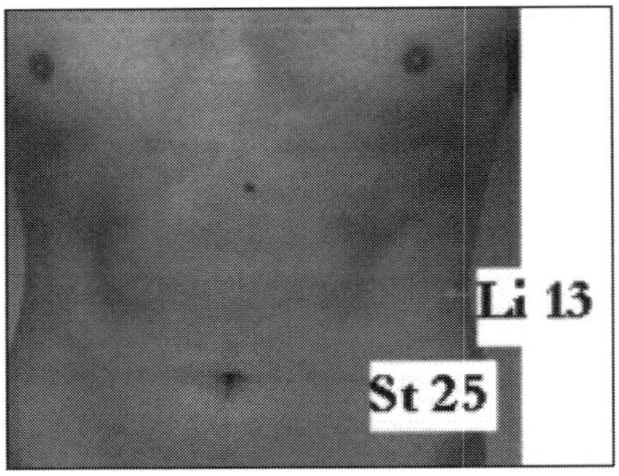

FIGURE 18.4

pain sometimes radiating to the side of the chest. This type also causes depression, panic, and, occasionally, acid reflux. The treatment is to adjust the liver energy and harmonize the stomach. The points are Ren 12 Zhong Wan San Li St 36 Zu San Li, Li

3 Tai Chong, Li 13 Zhang Men. Ren 12 and St 36 are used to adjust the stomach's functions and increase its energy and Li 3 will decrease the excesses of liver energy and create harmony in the stomach.

- **Chronic illness: Food stagnosis and indigestion.** The main symptoms are bloating, fullness in the stomach, bad smell in the mouth, poor appetite, sliding pulse, and tongue with white, wet, and thick coating. The treatment is to improve digestion and clear the food stoppage in the GI tract. For this, PC 6 Nei Guang, St 25 Tian Shu, St 36 Zu San Li, and St 44 Nei Ting are used.

JEFFREY'S TREATMENT

For Jeffrey, I used not only the points described above, but also points on the top of the head, such as Shi Sheng Chong and Du 20 Bai Hui, which can effectively decrease anxiety and panic attacks. After treatment, Jeffrey experienced immediate relief of his stomach aches, and as he gradually calmed down, the panic attacks subsided. I continued these treatments for five days, after which he had a complete recovery from the panic attacks. At this point he and I were able to have a reasonable discussion, which resulted in Jeffrey and his family moving to another state, where they lived in a house belonging to his sister-in-law. After two months he called to say he was rebuilding his life—he took his bar exam in this new state and now practices law there.

For anyone with emotional attacks plus a stomach ache, the most important thing to do initially is calm the person down and decrease the pain. Once this is accomplished, it is possible to have a substantive discussion about the root of the problem. This is very important in helping to completely relieve panic attacks so the problem-solving can begin. Once the cause of the problems that result in the stomach aches is determined, it is then possible to use acupuncture to help maximize a person's recovery.

TIPS FOR PERSONAL USE

- For an acute attack, you may use a heating pad on the stomach.
- Consistently press on acupressure point St 36 on outside of leg (see Figure 13.4). Acupressure the point with your thumb or knuckle, pressing on it with comfortable pressure.

19

Irritable Bowel Syndrome—IBS

LUCY'S ABDOMINAL PAINS

Lucy P. is a thirty-two-year-old student who came to me complaining of abdominal pain. She told me the pain is slow to come on. She feels it off and on and it can either be severe or mild. She also feels bloated and gaseous, and has constipation alternating with diarrhea, which produces mucus in the stool and is sometimes worse in the morning.

She generally feels mild depression, is shy and afraid to talk with people, and is unable to find a job. When she lived at home for five years after graduation, her parents encouraged her to go out and find employment, but her lack of communication skills made this impossible, so she decided to go back to school and earn a graduate degree in media communications. With graduation approaching, she began to feel nervous, knowing her parents expected her to get a job immediately after graduation. And she was depressed, experiencing insomnia, stomach aches, abdominal pain, and the bloating and diarrhea that sometimes turned to constipation. She was also vomiting and the pain and diarrhea she was experiencing interrupted her sleep and caused weight loss. She was frustrated with her condition, as were her parents, which is why she sought help from me.

A physical examination showed that Lucy had a soft abdomen, a normal bowel sound, no fever or chills, and a negative stool culture. I also sent her for a colonoscopy, which was negative as well. I determined that Lucy might have irritable bowel syndrome (IBS), a chronic gastrointestinal disorder of unknown cause, whose symptoms include the same abdominal cramping and pain, bloating, gassiness, and alternating bouts of diarrhea and constipation she was experiencing.

Unlike ulcerative colitis or Crohn's disease, IBS is not an inflammatory intestinal disease. It does not cause inflammation or changes in bowel tissues, and it does not increase the risk of colorectal cancer. In many cases, IBS may be attributed to diet, lifestyle, and stress. It can be very difficult to diagnose because IBS is a *diagnosis of exclusion.* A CT scan and laparotomy study may be needed, even a colonoscopy, to first rule out cancer, gastritis, peptic ulcer, or the like. After all these diseases have been eliminated, it is then possible to make a diagnosis of IBS—irritable bowel syndrome.

TREATMENTS IN WESTERN MEDICINE

People with irritable bowel syndrome should temporarily avoid all dairy products in order to rule out lactose intolerance, which sometimes mimics IBS. It is also necessary to avoid certain foods, such as the cruciferous vegetables—broccoli, Brussels sprouts, cabbage, and cauliflower—and beans as these can increase the bloating and gassiness. It may also help to increase the intake of fibers and try to decrease stress. If necessary, the doctor may prescribe antidepressant or antispasmodic medications, such as Bemote, Bentyl, and Lesin, or anti-diarrhea medication, such as Imodium. There are also some new medications that can probably help, such as tegaserod (brand name Zelnorm), used for the short-term treatment of IBS when constipation is the main symptom, and Lotronex, used for severe, chronic, diarrheapredominant IBS. This latter drug may, however, cause many undesirable side effects, including death in men, so this treatment is approved only for women—and then, as for all pharmaceutical drugs, with caution.

TREATMENTS IN TRADITIONAL CHINESE MEDICINE

The abdominal pain of this disorder is associated with the development of external disease and internal deficiency. Three types are associated with this condition.

- **Type 1 is excessive coldness.** Its main symptom is the abdominal pain, which becomes worse when the person drinks cold water. Also when the abdomen is exposed to cold in both the upper and

TABLE 19.1

POINTS	MERIDIAN NUMBER	CONDITIONS HELPED
1 Zhong Wan	Ren 12. See Figure 13.3	See Table 13.3
2 Guan Yuan	Ren 4. See Figure 21.2	See Table 21.1
3 Zu San U	St 36. See Figure 13.4	See Table 13.3
4 Gong Sun	Sp 4. See Figure 18.2	See Table 18.1

Please refer to the accompanying Figures (illustrations) for the locations of the points. And please note that these illustrations are for information only and may not show all the exact locations of the acupuncture points.

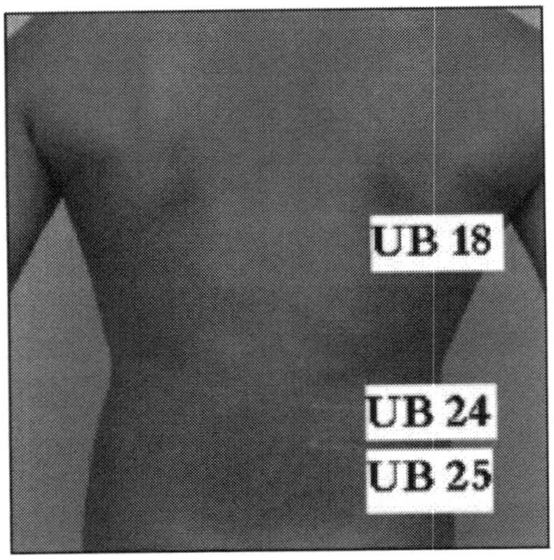

FIGURE 19.1

lower extremities, that leads to low energy. In this case, the large intestine has no pushing force and that triggers constipation; the person does not feel thirsty, however, and has long, cold urination. The principle of the treatment is to warm up the intestine and decrease the pain. The acupuncture points used are Ren 12 Zhong Wan, Ren 4 Guan Yuan, St 36 Zu San Li, and Sp 4 Gong Sun. The latter two can help decrease the coldness and improve the stomach movement, and St 36 and Sp 4 decrease the stomach ache and improve the spleen and stomach function.

- **Type 2 is excessive hotness of the abdomen.** This manifests itself in bloating, and in hardness and tenderness of the abdomen. The person craves cold water, becomes constipated, and experiences short, hot urination, and yellowish and dry coating of the tongue. The treatment for this condition is to eliminate the heat and treat the constipation. The acupuncture points are UB 25 Da Chang Shu, UB 24 Qi Hai Shu, St 37 Shang Ju Xu, LI 4 He Gu, LI 11 Qui Qi, St 44 Nei Ting, UB 24 and 25, and they are all very effective points to help bowel movements. LI 4 and LI 11 enhance the effectiveness of the rest of the points to improve bowel movements, so all these points together will increase pushing energy in the large intestine.

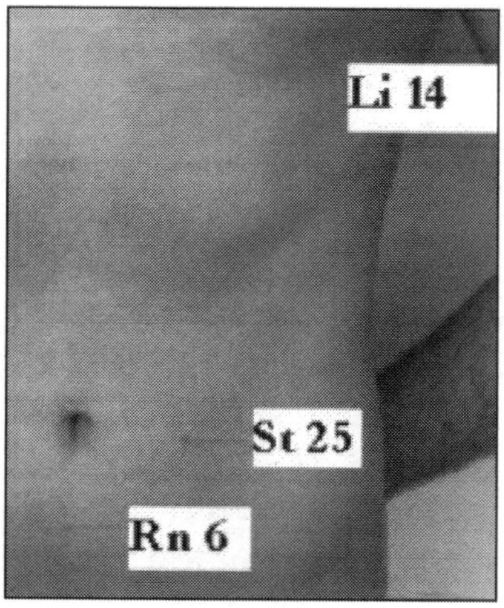

FIGURE 19.2

TABLE 19.2

POINTS	MERIDIAN NUMBER	CONDITIONS HELPED
1 Da Chang Shu	UB 25. See Figure 19.1	Low back pain, diarrhea constipation, muscular atrophy, pain, numbness and motor impairment of the lower extremities, sciatica
2 Qi Hai Shu	UB 24. See Figure 19.1	Low back pain, irregular menstruation, asthma
3 Shang Ju Xu	St 37. See Figure 19.3	Abdominal pain, diarrhea, dysentery, constipation, paralysis due to a stroke
4 He Gu	LI 4. See Figure 12.3	See Table 12.1
5 Qu Qi	Li 11. See Figure 12.2	See Table 12.2
6 Nei Ting	St 44. See Figure 18.2	See Table 18.1

Please refer to the accompanying Figures (illustrations) for the locations of the points. And please note that these illustrations are for information only and may not show all the exact locations of the acupuncture points.

- **Type 3** is excessive activity of the liver qi (energy) causing abdominal pain. The main symptoms are abdominal pain, anxiety, depression, and panic attacks, as well as a pain that radiates to the chest, and shooting pains down the side of the abdomen that feel better after a deep sigh. The pain becomes worse during a panic attack, depression, or periods of anxiety. The principal treatment for this type of IBS is to regulate the liver energy and decrease the abdominal pain, so the acupuncture points used for treatment are Liver UB 18 Gan Shu, Liver 3 Tai Cong, and Liver 14 Qi Meng. Since these points all are related to the liver, they will calm the hyperactivity of the liver energy, and improve the liver's function of regulating the stomach and the large intestine's movement and function. St 25 Tian Shu and St 36 Zu San Li are the important points that help make the necessary adjustment to the stomach and large intestine and decrease the diarrhea and constipation. GB 34 Yang Ling Quan and RN 6 Qi Hai improve the energy flow of the abdomen and decrease muscle spasms in the bowels and stomach. Taken together, all these points will help for this type of IBS.

TABLE 19.3

POINTS	MERIDIAN NUMBER	CONDITIONS HELPED
1 Can Shu	UB 18. See Figure 19.1	Backache, blurred vision, epilepsy, jaundice, mental disorders, night blindness, redness of the eye, spitting blood
2 Tai Cong	Li 3. See Figure 18.2	See Table 18.1
3 Qi Men	Li 14. See Figure 19.2	Acid regurgitation, depression, hiccups
4 Tian Shu	St 25. See Figure 19.2	Abdominal pain, constipation, diarrhea, dysentery, irregular menstruation, swelling
5 Yang Ling Quan	GB 34. See Figure 19.3	Bitter taste in the mouth, infantile convulsions, jaundice, numbness and pain of the lower extremities, swelling and pain of the knee, weakness, vomiting
6 Zu San U	St 36. See Figure 13.4	See Table 13.3

POINTS	MERIDIAN NUMBER	CONDITIONS HELPED
7 Qi Hai	RN 6. See Figure 19.2	Abdominal pain, nocturnal emission, impotence, hernia, swelling, diarrhea, dysentery, uterine bleeding, irregular menstruation, post–partum hemorrhage, constipation, asthma

Please refer to the accompanying Figures (illustrations) for the locations of the points. And please note that these illustrations are for information only and may not show all the exact locations of the acupuncture points.

LUCY'S TREATMENT

Lucy underwent treatment three times a week for five weeks, which greatly diminished her symptoms and gave her relief. I also prescribed some Chinese herbs for her constipation, and treated her depression with points on the top of her head (Shi Sheng Chong), which helped lessen her depression. Treating emotional disturbances is very important as it is one of the most effective remedies for IBS. Once Lucy's depression, anxiety, and panic attacks were brought under control, her IBS symptoms were greatly reduced.

TIPS FOR PERSONAL USE

- Take it easy. Emotional stress is very harmful for IBS.
- Focus on acupressure points St 36 and RN 6. Acupressure the points with your thumb or knuckle, pressing with comfortable pressure on the points; count to 20, then change to another point.

- Get deep massages and use a heating pad.

20

Alcohol Abuse

SAM'S DRINKING PROBLEM

Sam H., a sixty-two-year-old-man, is the owner and CEO of a large international company. He came to me complaining that his drinking had escalated owing to the hours he needed to keep in order to manage his multinational interests. He found it necessary to talk with people in many time zones, and his day often ran to fifteen or more hours. He initially started drinking during business hours only, to give him energy to cope with his long, stressful day, but soon extended his drinking to all hours of the day until he found he was consuming a bottle to a bottle and a half every day and was unable to cut down or quit his alcohol consumption. His customers began complaining that he was often incoherent on the phone, and he was afraid that his business, as well as his home life, would suffer irreparable damage due to his growing habit. When he discovered that alcohol had become both a physical and a psychological addiction, he knew he needed to back away from this.

CAUSES OF ALCOHOL ABUSE

Alcohol abuse, a dependence on drinking, is accompanied by one or more of the following problems.

- Failure to fulfill major work, school, and home responsibilities because of drinking.
- Drinking in situations that are physically dangerous, such as driving a car or operating machinery under the influence.
- Recurrent alcohol-related legal problems, such as being arrested for driving under the influence of alcohol, or physically hurting someone while drunk.
- Having problems with social or interpersonal relationship that are caused by the effects of alcohol.

Alcoholism is a severe pattern of drinking that includes the problems of alcohol abuse plus persistent drinking in spite of the obvious physical, mental, and social problems caused by alcohol. There are three major manifestations for alcoholism.

- Loss of control and inability to stop drinking once begun.
- Withdrawal symptoms associated with stopping, such as anxiety, nausea, shakiness, and sweating.
- Tolerance. Needing increased amounts of alcohol in order to maintain a *high.*

PROBLEMS RELATED TO ALCOHOL

Alcohol can cause many different problems, including physical, emotional, social, work-related, school, and financial difficulties. For health problems, the short-term effects include upset stomach, diarrhea, lack of coordination and judgment, headaches, and insomnia. The long-term health problems include high blood pressure and heart failure; liver damages, such as cancer, cirrhosis, and hepatitis; and problems related to the stomach, such as duodenal ulceritis, gastritis, peptic ulcer, or malnutrition. Insomnia often accompanies alcohol dependence, and there can be infections, plus loss of bone, kidney, muscle, and skin. Mental disorders include anxiety, depression, attention deficit, learning, memory deficiency, and mood swings; men can develop impotence and infertility. Social problems also plague alcoholics, including the loss of friends or jobs, child abuse, domestic violence, suppression of family members, and divorce.

TREATMENTS IN WESTERN MEDICINE

These are some of the numerous treatments for alcohol abuse and alcoholism.

- Counseling programs and rehabilitation centers.
- Support groups, including such twelve-step programs as Alcoholics Anonymous and Al-Anon for relatives and friends of alcoholics.
- Medicine—drugs and surgery. Although no magic pills to cure alcoholism have been developed yet, there are some drugs that can help reduce cravings as a first step to quitting.

- Aversion therapy.
- Alternative treatments, including exercise and vitamin therapy.

SAM'S TREATMENT WITH COUNSELING AND TRADITIONAL CHINESE MEDICINE—ACUPUNCTURE

From Sam's description of his problems, it was clear he could not stop drinking and had advanced to the withdrawal syndrome—when he stopped drinking, he said he felt nauseous, and had anxiety and sweats. He had also developed a tolerance for alcohol, which meant he had to drink more and more to feel drunk.

Sam and I discussed his treatment for alcoholism and I laid out the following points for him to consider.

- The most important thing for Sam was to admit and accept that alcohol abuse and alcoholism affect his work and his relationships with his family and colleagues. I made it very clear that the desire to stop was paramount to his success in conquering alcoholism, as it is with any addiction.
- I discussed the side effects and the consequences of the alcohol abuse, including liver deterioration, mental and social problems, and

all the many different side effects. Sam was shocked by the consequences of alcohol abuse and told me he was determined to stop drinking.

- Before undergoing treatment with me, I told Sam he had to agree to cooperate and stick to my treatment program, which was acupuncture three times a week for six to eight weeks. The withdrawal symptoms would last about this length of time, I told him. Sam was happy to agree to my terms and was very determined to follow my guidance. I also suggested he attend AA meetings, which he did, finding it easier to stick with a recovery program in the company of other alcoholics.

Acupuncture Treatments

TABLE 20.1

POINTS	MERIDIAN NUMBER	CONDITIONS HELPED
1 Sheng Men	Auricular. See Figure 20.1	
2 Sympathetic	Auricular. See Figure 20.1	
3 Subcortical	Auricular to treat generalized diseases in the subcortical region of the brain (below the cortex). See Figure 20.1	
4 Heart	Auricular to treat generalized heart disease. See Figure 20.1	
5 Stomach	Auricular to treat generalized stomach problems	
6 Endocrine	Auricular to treat generalized endocrine disorders. See Figure 20.1	

POINTS	MERIDIAN NUMBER	CONDITIONS HELPED
7 Throat	Auricular to treat generalized throat problems. See Figure 20.1	
8 Hunger/Thirst/Craving	Auricular to supress a craving for food, drugs, and alcohol. See Figure 20.1	

Please refer to the accompanying Figures (illustrations) for the locations of the points. And please note that these illustrations are for information only and may not show all the exact locations of the acupuncture points.

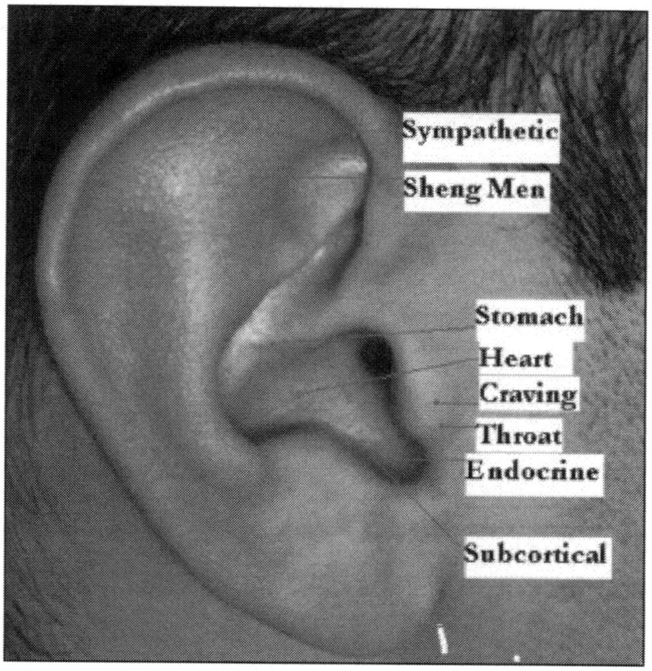

FIGURE 20.1

The number one group of the acupuncture points is the group of auricular (ear) acupuncture points, which include bilateral Sheng Men, sympathetic, subcortical, heart, stomach, endocrine, throat, and craving points. I inserted the needles in the above points and taped them so they would stay put. The inserted needles remain in the auricular points for one week, and if he craves a drink, Sam was asked to press those points for 1–2 minutes and to keep them pressed until the craving disappears. If he felt any withdrawal symptoms, such as anxiety or depression, he was also asked to press the subcortical, endocrine, and sympathetic points, which were pointed out to him, until all these symptoms disappeared.

For the body acupuncture, HT 7 Sheng Men, LI 4 He Gu, LI 11 Qu Qi, GB 20 Feng Chi, and Si Sheng Cong, the four points on the scalp.

The auricular points of Sheng Men, sympathetic, subcortical, and heart, can clean the mind and wake up the energy of the brain to improve mental function. The auricular points of stomach, endocrine, throat, and craving can suppress the craving sensation and decrease the activities of the mental-desire center. The body acupuncture point of HT 7 is a key point to improve mentality and make people feel calm, and relaxed, and it can help decrease the desire for alcohol consumption. The LI 4 and LI 11 both belong to the large intestine meridian and can help the body expel the wasted metabolics of alcohol. GB 20 can also help the HT 7 in improving the chain of thoughts and decreasing the craving of the alcohol, and the Si Sheng Cong, located on the top of the scalp, will clean the person's brain and help suppress the craving for alcohol. All of these points combined will decrease the craving for alcohol and improve the person's energy and mental functioning.

TABLE 20.2

POINTS	MERIDIAN NUMBER	CONDITIONS HELPED
1 Shen Men	HT 7. See Figure 20.2	Amnesia, cardiac pain, dementia, epilepsy, feverish sensation in the palm, insomnia, irritability, palpitations
2 He Gu	LI 4. See Figure 12.3	See Table 12.1
3 Qu Qi	LI 11. See Figure 12.2	See Table 12.2
4 Feng Chi	GB 20. See Figure 12.1	See Table 12.1
5 Si Sheng Cong	Ex–HN 1. See Figure 17.2	See Table 17.2

Please refer to the accompanying Figures (illustrations) for the locations of the points. And please note that these illustrations are for information only and may not show all the exact locations of the acupuncture points.

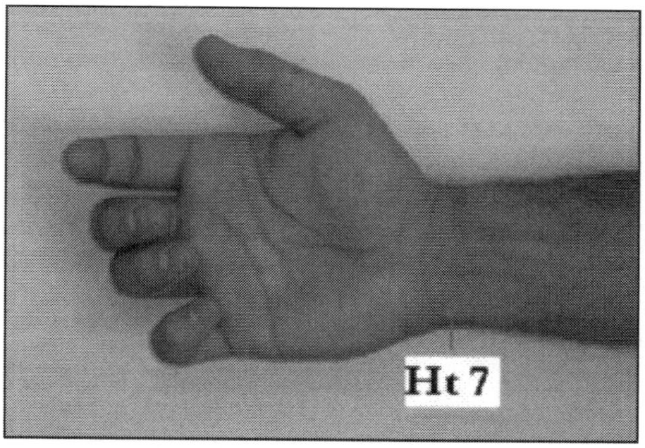

FIGURE 20.2

Sam continued seeing me, and after about two months in treatment, he completely stopped drinking. He told me his brain is functioning much better now, and his business and personal relationships are much improved as a result.

21

Weight Control

OBESITY

Susan W, a forty-five-year-old woman, came to me complaining of knee pain, which she had been experiencing for more than seven years, but which had become much worse in the past two months. I noted that, at about 5'6," she weighed in excess of 210lbs. and walked in an awkward position. She told me she liked to walk for exercise, and even run, but, because she was getting bigger and bigger, her knee pain was getting worse. She said she ate "very little" but was unable to get her weight down, and even walking caused pain as well as heart palpitations. She had high blood pressure and cholesterol. She claimed to have tried everything, including calorie control, exercise, and diet pills, but nothing had worked. Her clothes no longer fit and she was embarrassed to go to the gym and expose herself in exercise clothes.

CAUSES OF OBESITY AND OVERWEIGHT

Obesity is a chronic condition defined as an excess amount of body fat. The normal amount of body fat is between 25–30 percent in women and 18–24 percent in men. Anything over those percentages is considered obese.

Overweight is different from obesity. Overweight means having extra body weight from muscle, bone fat, and/or water. Obesity is having a high amount of extra body fat. The most useful measure of overweight and obesity is body mass index, which is based on height and weight and is used for adults, children, and teens.

The Reasons for Overweight and Obesity in Today's World

- Unbalanced energy in and out. In developed countries, the main cause of obesity is overeating; people ingest too many calories for their height and level of activity, so weight gain happens over time.
- Physical inactivity. Many Americans are not very physically active. One of the biggest reasons for this is spending too much time in front of computers and the television. A study finds that more than two hours of regular TV viewing per day has been linked to overweight and obesity.
- Other reasons include a dependence on cars instead of walking, and light physical demands at work and home. People who are inactive are more likely to gain weight because they do not burn up the calories they take in from food and drink.

- The environment. Our environment prevents a healthy lifestyle since there are not enough sidewalks for people to walk on and, since many people spend two or more hours commuting to their jobs, they do not have time for physical exercise.
- Lack of access to healthy foods or poor nutritional information.
- Genes and family history. Many people are obese because their parents were due to genes and bad habits relating to food and physical activity. There is definitely a link between genes and the environment, as children adopt the habits of their parents.
- Medical conditions, such as hypothyroidism and polycystic ovary syndrome.
- Medicines. Certain medicines, such as corticosteroids, prednisone, and antidepressants (Elavil, Neuront), can make people overeat.
- Depression and stress can lead to overeating as well.
- Age. As people age, they tend to lose muscle, especially if they become less active. Muscle loss slows down the rate at which the body burns calories. After age fifty, it is wise to reduce the number of calories consumed daily, otherwise it is easy to gain weight.
- Pregnancy. While it is normal to gain weight during pregnancy, many women retain this

weight even after the baby is born due to lack of activity and increased calorie intake.

- Lack of sleep. Studies have found that the less sleep people have, the more likely they are to be overweight or obese.
- Regular consumption of some high glycemic (GI) foods, such as refined carbohydrates and products made white flour or white sugar, can lead to a greater chance of developing a number of serious health problems, including cancer, cardiovascular disease, obesity, and type 2 diabetes.

THE GLYCEMIC INDEX

The glycemic index (GI) relates to the way your body's sugar levels respond to certain foods. Foods are given a rating from 0–100 on the glycemic index, with glucose in the highest position. High glycemic foods, such as simple, refined carbohydrate foods, will rapidly increase the body's sugar levels. Low glycemic foods will slowly increase the sugar levels in the body to sustain energy levels for longer periods of time. Low glycemic food is especially helpful in assisting those who want to lose weight. This is because an individual will feel less inclined to eat as energy is slowly being released into the bloodstream. Some health experts encourage using the glycemic index in conjunction with other meal programs to assist in managing diabetes and/or controlling weight. A diet that is primarily low glycemic is helpful in lowering blood cholesterol levels, controlling weight, maintaining energy, and promoting overall good health.

The glycemic index (GI) is a measure of the impact of carbohydrates on your blood glucose level. A test is performed using a sufficient quantity of a food to provide 50g of carbohydrates (referenced to white sugar or white bread). It considers the glycemic impact (GI/GL) which is critical for individuals with insulin resistance or carbohydrate sensitivity.

GI: low is 1–55; mid is 56–69; high is 70–100

Example: GI test requires 17oz carrots GI=47 low/mid

GL considers portion size (3oz) GL=5 low

Below is a list of glycemic index foods. It shows the food category and also the glycemic index for each particular food in that category.

TABLE 21.1. GI OF FOODS

BREADS	
White bread	70
Whole–meal bread	69
Pumpernickel	41
Dark rye	76
Sourdough	57
Heavy mixed grain	30–45
LEGUMES	

Lentils	28
Soybeans	18
Baked beans (canned)	48
BREAKFAST CEREALS	
Cornflakes	84
Rice Bubbles	82
Cheerios	83
Puffed Wheat	80
All Bran	42
Hot cereal	46
SNACK FOODS	
Mars Bar	65
Jelly beans	80
Chocolate bar	49
FRUITS	
Apple	38
Orange	44
Peach	42
Banana	55
Watermelon	72
DAIRY FOODS	
Milk, full fat	27
Milk, skim	32
Ice cream, full fat	61
Yogurt, low fat, fruit	33
SOFT AND SPORTS DRINKS	
Fanta	68
Gatorade	78

Source: www.healthyweightforum.org/eng/articles/glycemic-index/

MEDICAL RISKS AND DISEASES RELATED TO OBESITY AND OVERWEIGHT

The Centers for Disease Control (CDC) has defined obesity as being the *Number One* health epidemic in the U.S. Here are some statistics.

- Eighty percent of type 2 diabetes is obesity related, with 85 percent for kids.
- Seventy-two percent of cardiovascular disease is obesity related.
- Thirty percent of gallbladder surgeries are obesity related.
- Twenty-six percent of obese people have high blood pressure.

Risks that Obesity Poses to Good Health

Obesity can induce a substantial number of medical risks or diseases, as outlined below.

- Congestive heart failure, heart attacks, and heart disease. Many people who have coronary artery diseases and other heart related illness are afraid of physical activities and are stressed, so they do not perform physical exercise and very often eat junk food to reduce their stress. They put on weight and then, because of their increased weight, the heart has to pump more blood to the body, which increases the heart load, and which, in turn, can lead to congestive failure and a heart attack.

- High blood pressure. Obesity can induce high blood pressure, forcing the heart to pump more blood to the extremities, which increases the intensity in the arteries and makes the blood pressure go higher.
- Strokes. Deposits of fatty tissue in the blood vessels subsequently narrow the blood vessels and thereby decrease the blood supply to all the important organs. If the blood supply to the brain is blocked, this will cause a stroke.
- Type 2 diabetes. Overweight and obesity increase the resistance to the insulin contained in body tissue, which increases the work the pancreas has to do. Over time, this means the pancreas cannot secrete enough insulin, and a lack of insulin can cause low-density type 2 diabetes and high triglycerides.
- Increased cholesterol level. Because high-fat tissues supply a high amount of triglycerides and low-density lipoproteins, the bad cholesterol, they can cause heart attacks, hypertension, and similar.
- Cancer. Being obese raises the risk of breast, colon, endometrial, and gallbladder cancers.
- Osteoarthritis. Being overweight puts tremendous pressure on the low back, knee joints, and hip joints, and this can cause pain, as in Susan's case.
- Sleep apnea.

- Reproductive problems, such as infertility in women.
- Gallstones. Cholesterol can form gallstones, and these can cause abdominal or back pain.

BODY MASS INDEX

Overweight and obesity can be diagnosed by the body mass index (BMI). To determine this, first take your height and weight and then calculate your BMI using the following formula, or check the table (opposite).

A BMI of 18.5–24.9 is normal, below 18.5 is under normal weight, 25–29.9 is overweight, 30–39.9 is obese, and anything over 40 is morbidly obese.

BMI=weight (lb) x 703/height2 (in2)

BMI Categories

Underweight=<18.5	Normal weight=18.5–24.9
Overweight=25–29.9	Obesity=BMI of 30 or greater

TREATMENTS AND SURGERY IN WESTERN MEDICINE

Many people seek medical advice for weight loss. In mainstream Western medicine, the patient is sometimes prescribed anti-obesity medications to try and help with weight loss. There are two main medicines approved by the FDA for weight loss.

- Meridia, which sends signals to the brain to curb the appetite. It has, however, the side effects of raising blood pressure and pulse.
- Xenical, which reduces the absorption of fat and calories; it also blocks vitamins A, D, and K, which could cause mild side effects, such as loose stools.

There are also two kinds of weight loss surgery. The first is Roux-en-Y gastric bypass, the other is banded gastroplasty. Surgery usually has significant results, making the person lose between 40–50 pounds in a year. However, surgery might cause poor nutrition balance.

SUSAN'S TREATMENT IN TRADITIONAL CHINESE MEDICINE (TCM)

TABLE 21.2. BODY MASS INDEX (BMI 19–54)

To use the table, find the appropriate height in the left-hand column labeled Height. Move across to a given weight (in pounds). The number at the top of the column is the BMI at that height and weight. Pounds have been rounded off.

Source: National Heart Lung and Blood Institute www.nhlbi.nih.gov/guidelines/obesity/bmi_tbl.htm

BMI	19	20	21	22	23	24	25	26	27	28	29	30	31	32	33	34	35	36
Height (inches)	Body Weight (pounds)																	
58	91	96	100	105	110	115	119	124	129	134	138	143	148	153	158	162	167	172
59	94	99	104	109	114	119	124	128	133	138	143	148	153	158	163	168	173	178
60	97	102	107	112	118	123	128	133	138	143	148	153	158	163	168	174	179	184
61	100	106	111	116	122	127	132	137	143	148	153	158	164	169	174	180	185	190
62	104	109	115	120	126	131	136	142	147	153	158	164	169	175	180	186	191	196
63	107	113	118	124	130	135	141	146	152	158	163	169	175	180	186	191	197	203
64	110	116	122	128	134	140	145	151	157	163	169	174	180	186	192	197	204	209
65	114	120	126	132	138	144	150	156	162	168	174	180	186	192	198	204	210	216
66	118	124	130	136	142	148	155	161	167	173	179	186	192	198	204	210	216	223
67	121	127	134	140	146	153	159	166	172	178	185	191	198	204	211	217	223	230
68	125	131	138	144	151	158	164	171	177	184	190	197	203	210	216	223	230	236
69	128	135	142	149	155	162	169	176	182	189	196	203	209	216	223	230	236	243
70	132	139	146	153	160	167	174	181	188	195	202	209	216	222	229	236	243	250
71	136	143	150	157	165	172	179	186	193	200	208	215	222	229	236	243	250	257
72	140	147	154	162	169	177	184	191	199	206	213	221	228	235	242	250	258	265
73	144	151	159	166	174	182	189	197	204	212	219	227	235	242	250	257	265	272
74	148	155	163	171	179	186	194	202	210	218	225	233	241	249	256	264	272	280
75	152	160	168	176	184	192	200	208	216	224	232	240	248	256	264	272	279	287
76	156	164	172	180	189	197	205	213	221	230	238	246	254	263	271	279	287	295

BMI	37	38	39	40	41	42	43	44	45	46	47	48	49	50	51	52	53	54
Height (inches)	Body Weight (pounds)																	
58	177	181	186	191	196	201	205	210	215	220	224	229	234	239	244	248	253	258
59	183	188	193	198	203	208	212	217	222	227	232	237	242	247	252	257	262	267
60	189	194	199	204	209	215	220	225	230	235	240	245	250	255	261	266	271	276
61	195	201	206	211	217	222	227	232	238	243	248	254	259	264	269	275	280	285
62	202	207	213	218	224	229	235	240	246	251	256	262	267	273	278	284	289	295
63	208	214	220	225	231	237	242	248	254	259	265	270	278	282	287	293	299	304
64	215	221	227	232	238	244	250	256	262	267	273	279	285	291	296	302	308	314
65	222	228	234	240	246	252	258	264	270	276	282	288	294	300	306	312	318	324
66	229	235	241	247	253	260	266	272	278	284	291	297	303	309	315	322	328	334
67	236	242	249	255	261	268	274	280	287	293	299	306	312	319	325	331	338	344
68	243	249	256	262	269	276	282	289	295	302	308	315	322	328	335	341	348	354
69	250	257	263	270	277	284	291	297	304	311	318	324	331	338	345	351	358	365
70	257	264	271	278	285	292	299	306	313	320	327	334	341	348	355	362	369	376
71	265	272	279	286	293	301	308	315	322	329	338	343	351	358	365	372	379	386
72	272	279	287	294	302	309	316	324	331	338	346	353	361	368	375	383	390	397
73	280	288	295	302	310	318	325	333	340	348	355	363	371	378	386	393	401	408
74	287	295	303	311	319	326	334	342	350	358	365	373	381	389	396	404	412	420
75	295	303	311	319	327	335	343	351	359	367	375	383	391	399	407	415	423	431
76	304	312	320	328	336	344	353	361	369	377	385	394	402	410	418	426	435	443

As I usually do for weight control, I used the following programs together.

I first ruled out any medical illness that might have caused her obesity. She was screened for polycystic ovary syndrome and checked for hypothyroidism and/or Cushing's syndrome. All tests came back normal.

Acupuncture

TABLE 21.3

POINTS	MERIDIAN NUMBER	CONDITIONS HELPED
1 Liang Qiu	St 34. See Figure 21.1	Gastric pain, motor impairment of the lower extremities, pain and numbness of the knee
2 Gong Sun	Sp 4. See Figure 21.1	Gastric pain, vomiting, abdominal pain and distension, diarrhea, dysentery
3 Zhong WanRen	Ren 12. See Figure 21.2	Stomach ache, abdominal distention, nausea, vomiting, acid regurgitation, diarrhea, dysentery, jaundice, indigestion, insomnia
4 Guang YuanRen	Ren 4. See Figure 21.2	Lower abdominal pain, indigestion, diarrhea, nocturnal emission, frequency of urination, retention of urine, hernia, irregular menstruation, postpartum hemorrhage

Please refer to the accompanying Figures (illustrations) for the locations of the points. And please note that these illustrations are for information only and may not show all the exact locations of the acupuncture points.

I combined body acupuncture with auricular (ear) acupuncture points.

- For the body, the most important points are St 34, Liang Qiu points and Sp 4, Gong Sun. Liang Qiu points belong to the stomach meridian and can inhibit stomach activity and make the food absorption slower and decrease the appetite. Gong Sun SP 4 is a point of the spleen, which can increase the body's metabolism and decrease the appetite, too. Ren 12 Zhong Wan and Ren 3 Guang Yuan are local points adjacent to the stomach and intestine, they directly affect and facilitate the bowel movement, therefore, inhibit the absorption of the food in the GI system.

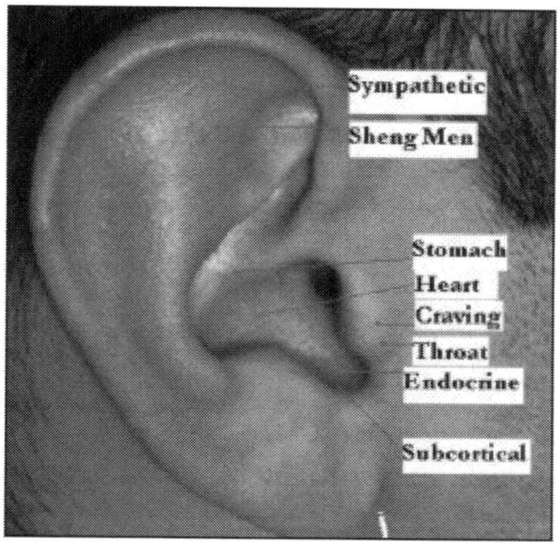

FIGURE 21.1

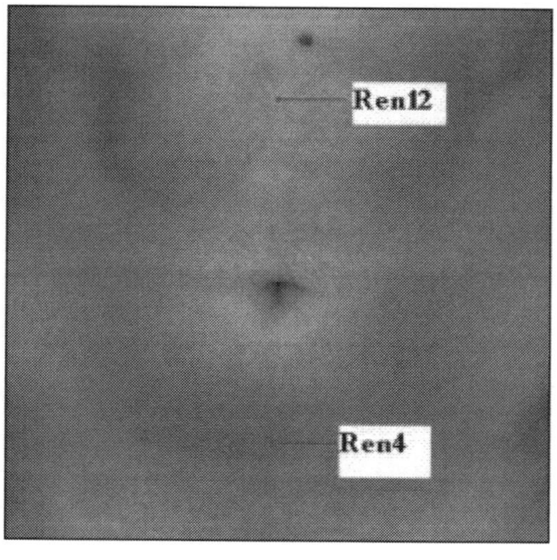

FIGURE 21.2

- Auricular needles are the most important part of a weight loss program. I chose the points of spleen, stomach, liver, small intestine, and Sheng Meng. These points can inhibit stomach activity, slow the absorption of nutrition from food in the stomach and small intestine and also improve energy and decrease stress and depression.

I taped the needles to Susan ears and advised her to press them to lessen her craving for food when she was feeling hungry. The points on the liver, endocrine, and Sheng Meng may reduce stress and anxiety, and the points of spleen, stomach, and small intestine decrease the craving sensation. For those who fear needles, it is possible to substitute vegetable or plastic seeds in place of the needles, and, generally speaking, they will have the same effect.

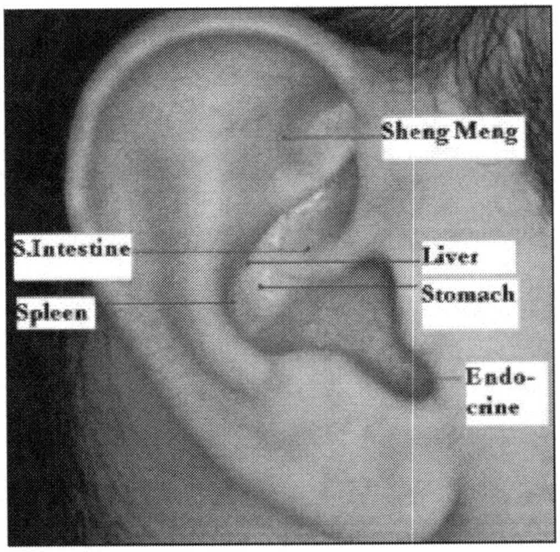

FIGURE 21.3

Diet Program

Diet is the most important and the most difficult part of entire weight loss program. The principal is, ***You must eat less than the calories you burn.***

The following are the most crucial points to follow.

- Eat a healthy and a good breakfast. You may eat as much healthy food as you like for breakfast. I do not suggest skipping breakfast because you need breakfast to supply an entire day's energy.
- Have a moderate meal at lunch to maintain necessary energy for afternoon.
- Eat a minimum dinner or no dinner. Most Americans do the opposite. They eat no breakfast, eat a moderate lunch, and finish the day with a huge dinner because they think they deserve the banquet after a day of hard work. However, they do not understand that they can burn the calories they take in during the daytime due to their work. Most people watch television after dinner or engage in some other activity that burns few, if any, calories, so the foods eaten at dinner, which have all night to be digested, mostly turn to fat. Turning around the way you eat can cause significant weight loss, with breakfast as the largest meal, and dinner small or non-existent.
- As previously described, eat low glycemic-index food.

Additional Elements of the Diet Program

Chinese herbal program. I usually prescribe herbs to improve bowel movements and loosen the bowels. This hastens the food through the system faster than usual and diminishes the time it's there to be absorbed as fat.

Nutritional supplements. There are thousands of nutritional supplements on the market. After careful selection, I chose four supplements for my patients.

1. Transitions Carbohydrate Absorption Inhibitor (CAI). CAI inhibits the enzymes that normally break down starch into glucose in the small intestine. As a result, the absorption of glucose from carbohydrate-rich foods, such as bread, potatoes, rice, and pasta is limited. The active ingredient of CAI, wheat amylase inhibitor, has the advantage of maximum effectiveness in small amounts.
2. Transitions Conjugated Linoleic Acid (CLA) Caffeine Free. This is ideal for those who have lost weight or are losing weight and want the extra support to keep it off. Transitions CLA Caffeine Free contains natural ingredients that can help redistribute fat to fat-burning muscle tissue to assist in promoting lean muscle mass and decreasing the amount of fat stored in your body.
3. Transitions Fat Conversion Inhibitor (FCI). This helps reduce the number of calories being con-

verted to fat, assists in maintaining normal blood sugar levels, and can decrease appetite. It contains the natural ingredient *Garcinia Cambogia* that inhibits the fat conversion process in your body's cells and promotes more effective burning of calories. *Garcinia Cambogia* also increases serotonin levels, which controls your appetite, putting you in control. Transitions FCI contains additional natural ingredients that effectively promote weight loss: *Gymnema Sylvestre* is a natural herb that can help maintain blood sugar levels and reduce cravings for sweets. Chromium is an essential trace mineral that promotes normal glucose uptake by the cells. This process aids in the maintenance of blood sugar levels and ultimately helps maintain your energy level and decrease your cravings.

4. Transitions Thermochrome with Advantra Z and South African *Hoodia Gordonii.* This is a unique blend of herbs, extracts, and vitamins that promises to provide you with calorie burning (thermogenesis), fat burning (lipolysis), and appetite suppression all in one product. Typically, when you restrict calories/intake, your body stops working as hard and your metabolism slows down. Transition Thermochrome allows you to restrict calories while maintaining your metabolism and increasing the burning of body fat for fuel. Termochrome also has Advantra Z, which may help to control your appetite.

Physical Activity

I encourage my patients to do physical exercise for forty-five minutes to an hour, six days a week. If they don't exercise, they won't be able to burn the calories they eat. Susan liked to run, but I advised her to give up running and instead swim and work out on a stationary bicycle, as these activities do not have a negative impact on the knees and hip joints. They are also very good exercises for the entire body, especially all the other joints. Susan now swims and bicycles about one hour a day, six days a week.

THE RESULTS OF SUSAN'S TCM TREATMENT

After two months of sticking to her program, Susan lost fourteen pounds. To prevent infection, her auricular needles were changed once a week. She continued to take the Chinese herbs and the nutritional supplements, and kept up her diet and physical activity program. After six months, she had lost almost forty pounds and no longer needed the auricular needles. As expected, after she lost weight, her knee pain was much improved.

TIPS TO USE AT HOME OR OFFICE

- The key is the dinner. If you eat very little dinner, or no dinner, you will lose weight very soon.

- Healthy eating habits primarily utilize foods on the low glycemic diet. A primarily low glycemic diet is helpful in lowering blood cholesterol levels, controlling weight, maintaining energy, and promoting overall good health. Regular consumption of certain high-glycemic (GI) foods can lead to a greater chance of developing serious health problems, including obesity, cancer, cardiovascular disease, and type 2 diabetes.
- The acupuncture and the nutritional supplements will greatly decrease your appetite.
- Exercise will help you burn more calories. The following ideas will help you do more exercise without spending more time doing them.

  * Always park your car far away from the shopping center or any place you go.

  * Try to walk upstairs and downstairs without taking an elevator.

  * Always hold in your abdomen while you are sitting in your chair.

  * Always walk somewhere if you do not have to drive.

  * If you like to use walking as an exercise, attach a 5lb weight to each calf muscle. You will achieve much greater success in the same amount of time.
- For more information, please visit: www.win.niddk .nih.gov/publica-tions/myths.htm

22

Headaches

JOAN'S TEENAGE HEADACHES

Joan T., a sixteen-year-old schoolgirl, was brought to me by her mother because the girl had been experiencing headaches since she was twelve and first got her period. Her headaches were so severe that four or five days a week during her period she was often unable to go to school. These headaches manifested themselves on both temporal regions of her head and also caused severe pain to the left eye. Because of the pain's severity, the headaches were interfering with her schoolwork. Joan had to call her mother several days a week to pick her up from school, which, for several years made it necessary for the mother to quit her job and begin to home school Joan.

At sixteen, Joan returned to school as a junior because she needed to start preparing for college entrance exams, as well as apply to colleges. Soon afterward, the pain had grown so severe that Joan was sleeping poorly and was extremely stressed, which often resulted in tears and depression, and, in turn, made her eat too much, causing a large weight gain. Her mother had taken her to many doctors over the years, and she had been prescribed a variety of drugs, but nothing seemed to help the migraines. Her SAT exams were coming up in two months when the mother finally brought her to me for evaluation.

A physical examination showed Joan to be a slightly obese young girl, very depressed, and stressed. She spoke in a low tone; did not like light, and felt pain when her temporal area and the back of her scalp, the occipital area, were touched.

TYPES OF HEADACHES

I considered that Joan might have one of the following three types of primary headaches: tension, cluster, or migraine. She could also have a mix of two or three of them.

Tension Headaches

This is the most common type of chronic and frequent headaches. The symptoms include steady pain on both sides of the head with a feeling of pressure and tightness around the head, as if a band was put tightly around it. The pain radiates from the back, eyes, neck, or other parts of the body, and usually increases over period of hours. As it worsens, it can develop a pulsating quality.

Source: http://health.stateuniversity.com/pages/1498/Tension-Headache.html

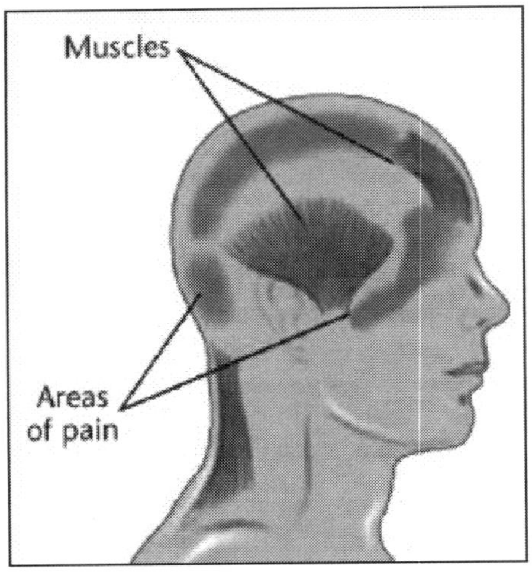

FIGURE 22.1

Cluster Headaches

This type of headache is often described as a sharp penetrating or burning sensation in one eye where the person feels as if somebody had punched her or his eye. The pain comes on suddenly, without warning, and within a few minutes, excruciating pain develops that can be so severe some women report it is even worse than childbirth. People with cluster headaches often appear restless. These headaches usually last about two to twelve weeks, though some chronic cluster headaches may continue for more than a year. They sometimes go with seasonal change.

Source: http://en.wikipedia.org/wiki/Cluster_headache

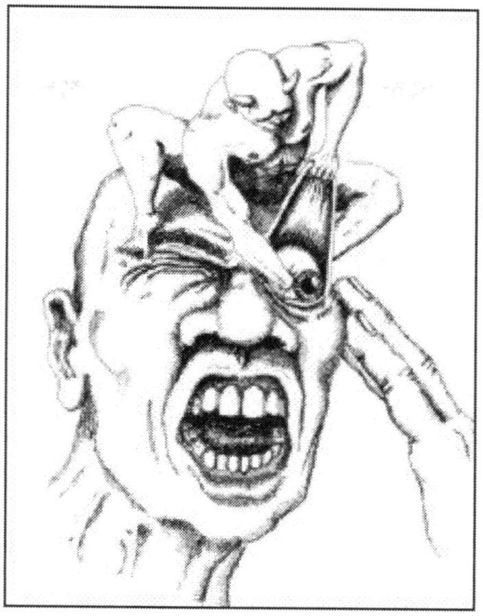

FIGURE 22.2

Migraine Headaches

A migraine headache is a throbbing or pulsating headache that is often on one side of the head and is associated with nausea and vomiting, sensitivity to light, sound, and smell, with sleep disruption and depression. These attacks are very often recurrent and do not change with age, sometimes developing into chronic migraine headaches.

There are two types of migraine headaches: migraine with aura and migraine without aura. Most auras are visual and are described as bright shining light around objects or at the edges of the field of vision, hallucinations, or zigzag lines with a wave image. Some people may experience dizziness, motor weakness, numbness, speech or language abnormalities, temporary vision loss, tingling, or vertigo.

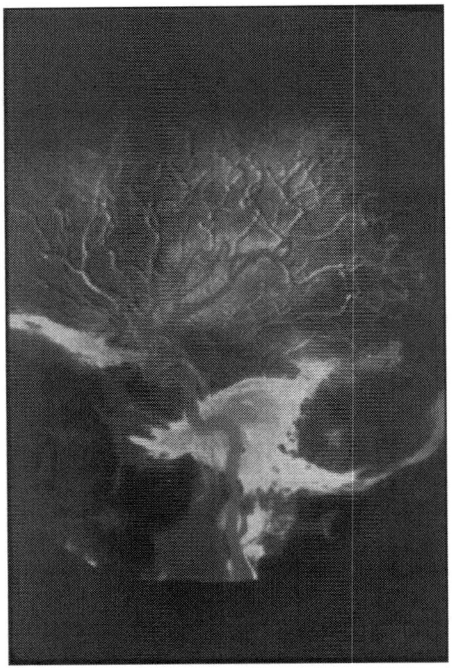

FIGURE 22.3. An MRI of a Migraine.

Source: bfnorth.com

CAUSES OF THE THREE TYPES OF HEADACHES

- The causes of tension headaches are usually stress, muscular tension, gouty arthritis on the neck or spine, postural changes, vascular dilation, protracted coughing or sneezing, fever and depression, or temporal mandibular joint disorder.
- The cause of cluster headaches is unknown. However, cluster headaches are known to be triggered by alcohol, nitroglycerin, or similar drugs.
- The cause of migraine headaches is also unknown. There may be a family history of the disorder, or

a migraine can be triggered by many stimulants: alcohol, altitude, color, contrasting pattern, exertion, food, hormonal change, hunger, lack of sleep, medicine, perfume, stress, and weather.

TREATMENTS IN WESTERN MEDICINE

From the Western medicine point of view, there are many different kinds of medications to treat headaches. For example, Topamax and Imitrex are used for migraine headaches with some successful result. However, when beta blockers, antiseizure medication, calcium channel blockers, tricyclic antidepressants, and analgesics, such as aspirin, ibuprofen, and acetaminophen, are used to treat migraine, cluster, or tension headaches, they cannot provide significant improvement for any of these headaches. Therefore, more and more people are starting to look for alternative treatments, and acupuncture is one of the best.

TREATMENTS IN TRADITIONAL CHINESE MEDICINE

Chinese medicine classifies headaches in two categories.

External Wind Attack Headaches

These headaches are caused by external factors, such as wind cold and wind heat. The headaches are usually characterized by an acute onset and a very severe and constant attack.

- **Wind cold.** This causes periodic attacks, where the pain always is connected with the neck and upper back and an aversion to wind and cold. The head feels heavy, as if a tight band is wrapped around it. The person does not feel thirsty, and has a thin, white coating on the tongue, and a floating pulse.
- **Wind heat.** This type feels like a headache expanding from inside the head, accompanied by fever and an aversion to heat and wind, with a reddish face and eyes. The person feels thirsty, has constipation, yellowish urine, a red tongue body, with yellow coating on the tongue, and a floating pulse.

Internal Organ Dysfunction Headaches

These headaches are usually of slow onset with mild pain and sometimes the feeling of emptiness within the head. When people are stressed and overworked, the pain will be worse. The pain is on and off and usually lasts for a long time.

The Meridians

According to traditional Chinese medicine, the head, the face, and also the liver are where all six yang meridians go. Since these meridians go up to the top of the head, headaches can be diagnosed based on the meridian distribution. If you know the meridian distribution, it will be easier to make a clear diagnosis and treatment.

- Tai Yang (Urinary Bladder) meridian headache. This is usually located at the top of the head, or the back of the head, and is connected to the neck.
- Yang Ming (Large Intestine) meridian headache: This is usually in the front of the head—on the forehead—and includes the upper portion of the eye.
- Shao Yang (Gallbladder) meridian headache: This is usually on both temporal areas and radiates to the ear.
- Jue Ying (Liver) meridian headache: This is usually on the top of the head, sometimes connecting to the eyes and forehead.

Acupuncture for Headaches

I first ask my patient the location of the headache and its severity in order to find out which internal organ shows dysfunction. I next ask about the accompanying symptoms in order to differentiate the wind cold from the wind heat.

For Tai Yang (Urinary Bladder) meridian headache on the top of the head and back of the neck, the following are used: GB 20 Feng Chi, DU 16 Feng Fu, DU 19 Hou Ding, UB 9 Yu Zhen, UB 60 Kun Run, and SI 3 Hou Xi.

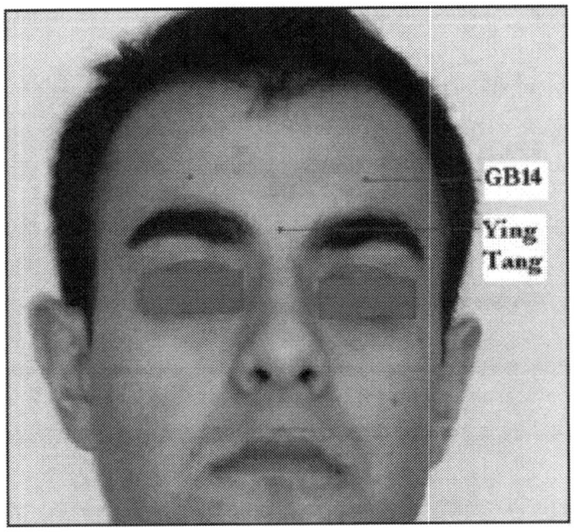

FIGURE 22.4

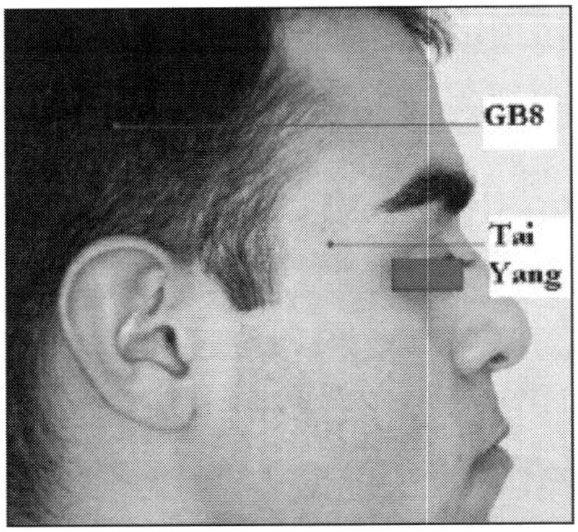

FIGURE 22.5

The Yang Ming (Large Intestine) meridian headache centers on the front of the head, the forehead, including the upper portion of the eye. The acupuncture points are Yin Tang and Tai Yang (Extraordinary Points), Lu 7 Lie Que, LI 4 He Gu, and GB 14 Yang Bai.

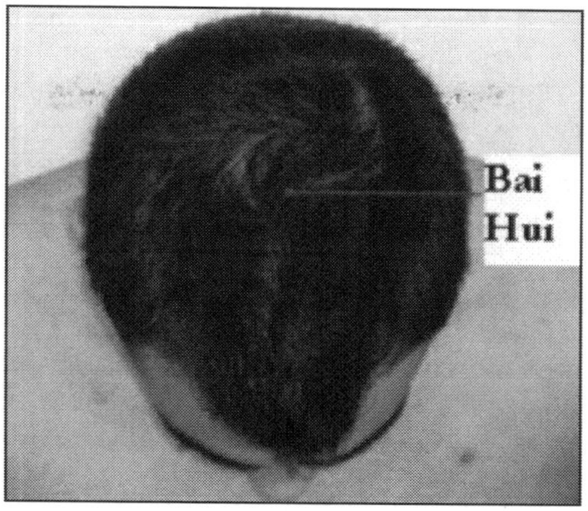

FIGURE 22.6

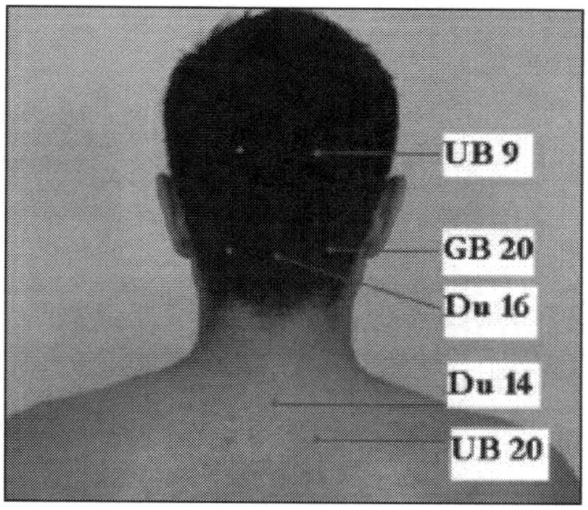

FIGURE 22.7

The Shao Yang (Gallbladder) meridian headache is usually on the bilateral temporal area and radiates to the ear. The following points are chosen: GB 20 Feng Chi, Extraordinary Point 1 Tai Yang, SJ 5 Wai Guan, ST 8 Tao Wei, and GB 38 Yang Fu, and GB 39 Jue Gu.

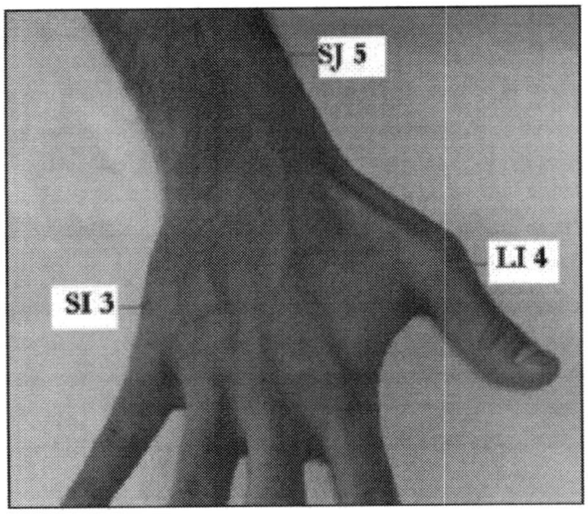

FIGURE 22.8

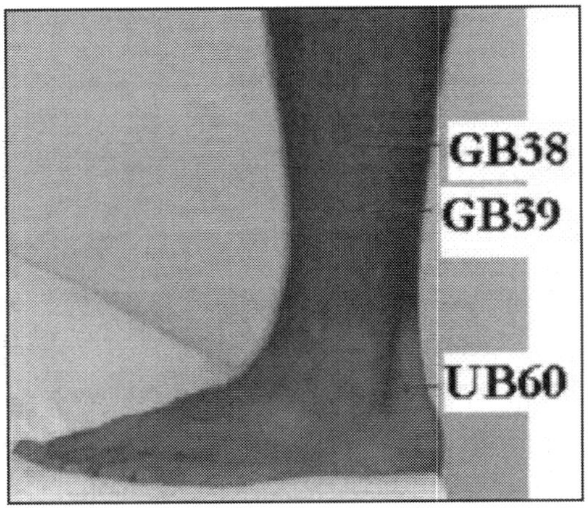

FIGURE 22.9

TABLE 22.1

POINTS	MERIDIAN NUMBER	CONDITIONS HELPED
1 Feng Chi	Gallbladder 20. See Figure 22.7	Headaches, vertigo, insomnia, pain and stiffness of the neck, blurred vision, glaucoma, red and painful eyes, tinnitus, convulsion, epilepsy, infantile convulsions, common cold, nasal obstruction

POINTS	MERIDIAN NUMBER	CONDITIONS HELPED
2 Feng Fu	DU 16. See Figure 22.7	Headaches, neck rigidity, blurred vision, nosebleed, sore throat, mental disorders
3 Hou Ding	DU 19. See Figure 22.7	Headaches, vertigo, epilepsy
4 Yu Zhen	Urinary Bladder 9. See Figure 22.7	Headaches, neck pain, dizziness, nasal obstruction
5 Kun Lun	Urinary Bladder 60. See Figure 22.9	Headaches, blurred vision, neck rigidity, pain in the shoulder, back, and arm, swelling and heel pain, difficult labor, epilepsy
6 Hou Xi	Small Intestine 3. See Figure 22.8	Pain and rigidity of the neck, tinnitus, deafness, sore throat, acute lumbar sprain, night sweat, fever, numbness of the finger and shoulder, elbow pain

Please refer to the accompanying Figures (illustrations) for the locations of the points. And please note that these illustrations are for information only and may not show all the exact locations of the acupuncture points.

TABLE 22.2

POINTS	MERIDIAN NUMBER	CONDITIONS HELPED
1 Yin Tang	Extraordinary Point. See Figure 22.4	Headaches, head heaviness, infantile convulsion, frontal headaches, insomnia
2 Tai Yang	Extraordinary Point. See Figure 22.5	Headaches, eye diseases, off–center deviation of the eyes and mouth
3 Lie Que	Lung 7. See Figure 12.2	Cough, pain in the chest, asthma, sore throat, spasmodic pain of the elbow and arm

POINTS	MERIDIAN NUMBER	CONDITIONS HELPED
4 He Gu	Large Intestine 4. See Figure 12.3	Headaches, pain in the neck, redness, swelling, and pain of the eye, nosebleed, nasal obstruction, toothache, deafness, swelling of the face, sore throat, facial paralysis, abdominal pain, dysentery, constipation, delayed labor, pain, weakness, and motor impairment of the upper limbs
5 Yang Bai	Gall Bladder 14. See Figure 22.4	Headaches, pain in the orbital ridge, eye pain, vertigo, twitching of the eyelids, tearing

Please refer to the accompanying Figures (illustrations) for the locations of the points. And please note that these illustrations are for information only and may not show all the exact locations of the acupuncture points.

TABLE 22.3

POINTS	MERIDIAN NUMBER	CONDITIONS HELPED
1 Feng Chi	Gallbladder 20. See Figure 22.7	Headaches, vertigo, insomnia, neck pain and stiffness, blurred vision, glaucoma, pink and painful eyes, tinnitus, convulsions, epilepsy, infantile convulsion, febrile (fever) diseases, common cold, nasal obstruction, runny nose
2 Tai Yang	Extraordinary Point. See Figure 22.5	Headaches, eye diseases, off–center deviation of the eyes and mouth
3 Wai Guan	San Jiao 5. See Figure 22.8	Fever, headaches, cheek and neck pain, deafness, tinnitus, elbow and arm pain, hand tremor

POINTS	MERIDIAN NUMBER	CONDITIONS HELPED
4 Tou Wei	Stomach 8. See Figure 22.10	Headaches, blurred vision, eye pain, excessive tears
5 Yang Fu	Gallbladder 38. See Figure 22.9	Migraines
6 Jue Gu	Gallbladder 39. See Figure 22.9	Apoplexy, neck pain muscular atrophy of the lower limbs, spastic pain of the leg

Please refer to the accompanying Figures (illustrations) for the locations of the points. And please note that these illustrations are for information only and may not show all the exact locations of the acupuncture points.

For Jue Ying (Liver) meridian headache, the pain is usually on the top of the head and it often connects to the eyes and forehead. The following points are chosen: Du 20 Bai Hui, Liv 3 Tai Chong, and Lung 7 Lie Que.

TABLE 22.4

POINTS	MERIDIAN NUMBER	CONDITIONS HELPED
1 Bai Hui	Du 20. See Figure 22.6	Headaches, vertigo, tinnitus, nasal obstruction, coma, mental disorders, prolapse of the rectum and the uterus
2 Tai Chong	Liv 3. See Figure 18.2	Headaches, dizziness, insomnia, congestion, swelling and pain of the eye, depression, infantile convulsions, uterine bleeding, hernia, retention of urine, epilepsy
3 Lie Que	Lung 7. See Figure 12.2	Headaches, migraine, neck stiffness, cough, asthma, sore throat, facial paralysis, toothache, wrist pain and weakness

Please refer to the accompanying Figures (illustrations) for the locations of the points. And please note that these illustrations are for information only and may not show all the exact locations of the acupuncture points.

If the above symptoms are accompanied with the wind cold or wind heat signs, I add the following points:

For Wind Cold: GB 20 Feng Chi, Extraordinary Point Tai Yang, St 8 Tou Wei, GB 8 Shuai Gu, UB 12 Feng Meng, and UB 60 Kun Lun.

TABLE 22.5

POINTS	MERIDIAN NUMBER	CONDITIONS HELPED
1 Feng Chi	Gallbladder 20. See Figure 22.7	Headaches, dizziness, insomnia, neck pain and stiffness, blurred vision, glaucoma, pink and painful eyes, tinnitus, convulsions, epilepsy, infantile convulsion, febrile (fever) diseases, common cold, nasal obstruction, runny nose
2 Tai Yang	Extraordinary Point. See Figure 22.5	Headaches, eye diseases, off–center deviation of the eyes and mouth
3 Tou Wei	Stomach 8. See Figure 22.10	Headaches, blurred vision, eye pain, excessive tears
4 Shuai Gu	Gallbladder 8. See Figure 22.5	Migraines, vertigo, vomiting, infantile convulsions
5 Feng Meng	Urinary Bladder 12. See Figure 22.11	Common cold, cough, fever and headaches, neck rigidity, back pain
6 Kun Lun	Urinary Bladder 60. See Figure 22.9	Headaches, blurred vision, neck rigidity, pain in the shoulder, back, and arm, swelling and heel pain, difficult labor, epilepsy

Please refer to the accompanying Figures (illustrations) for the locations of the points. And please note that these illustrations are for information only and may not show all the exact locations of the acupuncture points.

For Wind Heat: GB 20 Feng Chi, Tai Yang, St 8 Tou Wei, GB 8 Shuai Gu, Du 14 Da Zhui, and SJ 5 Wai Guan.

TABLE 22.6

POINTS	MERIDIAN NUMBER	CONDITIONS HELPED
1 Feng Chi	Gallbladder 20. See Figure 22.7	Headaches, vertigo, insomnia, neck pain and stiffness, blurred vision, glaucoma, pink and painful eyes, tinnitus, convulsions, epilepsy, infantile convulsion, febrile (fever) diseases, common cold, nasal obstruction, runny nose
2 Tai Yang	Extraordinary Point. See Figure 22.5	Headaches, eye diseases, deviation of eyes and mouth
3 Tou Wei	Stomach 8. See Figure 22.10	Headaches, blurred vision, eye pain, excessive tears
4 Shuai Gu	Gallbladder 8. See Figure 22.5	Migraines, vertigo (dizziness), vomiting, infantile convulsions
5 Da Zhui	Du 14. See Figure 22.7	Neck pain and rigidity, malaria, fever, epilepsy, cough, asthma, common cold, back pain and stiffness
6 Wai Guan	San Jiao 5. See Figure 22.8	Febrile (fever) diseases, headaches, cheek pain, neck sprain, elbow, arm, and finger pain, hand tremors, abdominal pain

Please refer to the accompanying Figures (illustrations) for the locations of the points. And please note that these illustrations are for information only and may not show all the exact locations of the acupuncture points.

JOAN'S TREATMENT

Joan's headaches were very complicated. From the Western medicine point of view, her headaches belonged to the migraine category. However, her headaches were always triggered by nerve pain in the back of the head and worsened with her hormonal changes and menstruation. She had four to five attacks a week, and every time she had the nerve pain or a hormonal change, her headache symptoms would get worse.

After I made a clear diagnosis, I first used GB 20, DU 16, and Du 20 Bai Hui, and then Extraordinary points Tai Yang and LI 4 He Gu. I gave Joan this treatment three times a week for about two months and also injected her with cortisone to block the left and right nerve pain in the back of her head. Her headaches improved a great deal after this treatment and she was able to take her SATs and apply for college. She was accepted by Boston College and when I followed up on her two years later, her mother reported that Joan had no more major headache attacks. She survived her college study and her mother is very thankful to me.

ACUPRESSURE TIPS TO USE AT HOME OR OFFICE

- If you have a headache, be specific as to the site of the headache and identify if you have a Tai Yang, Yang Ming, Shao Yang, or Jue Ying headache.
- After you identify the site of the headache, then try to locate the points by following the tables and illustrations above.
- Acupressure the points with your knuckle, press with comfortable pressure on the points, count 20, and then change to another point. You should work any symmetric points at the same time.
- Since the acupressure points are located mainly on your head, use the head points as the major acupressure points. You may ask your friends or family members to help you with moderate acupressure.

23

Insomnia

ALICE'S SLEEPING DIFFICULTIES

Alice E, a forty-five-year-old woman, came to me complaining of insomnia. She had the same difficulty falling asleep, especially after experiencing stress, that she'd had at college on the nights before exams. She would lie in her bed, staring at the ceiling, and not fall asleep. If she was lucky enough to doze off, she would wake up frequently, even at the slightest noise. She had experienced this problem for about ten years, but recently the problem had escalated, owing to her marital situation. Her husband, the CEO of a large company, had quit his job because he would not fly from New York to Houston each Monday, then return to New York each weekend. He had managed this schedule for two years, but it had become too burdensome to him, hence his decision to quit. Tough he sent out many resumes each week, his job search had produced no results, and the family's financial situation had become difficult over the six months her husband had been unemployed. For the last two or three months, she could only sleep an hour or two each night, owing to stress, and this caused her difficulty during the day, as she found it hard to concentrate on any issue. This sleep deprivation impaired her memory, her social interactions, and her motor coordination, which caused problems with her driving. It was at this point she consulted me.

TYPES AND CAUSES OF INSOMNIA

Insomnia is a symptom, not a disease. It is defined as difficulty in initiating, or maintaining, sleep—or both. It is due to an inadequate quality or quantity of sleep. Most adults have experienced insomnia or sleeplessness at one time or another in their lives.

Insomnia can be classified based on the duration of the problem:

- Transient insomnia. These symptoms last less than one week.
- Short-term insomnia. Symptoms last between one and three weeks.
- Chronic insomnia. Symptoms last longer than three weeks.

Most Common Reasons for Insomnia

- Stress. Many people experience stress from the environment, including that caused by life, work, family, and the like. This keeps them thinking about the stress and trying to deal with it, which makes falling asleep extremely difficult.
- Anxiety. Everyday activity and anxiety, or severe anxiety disorder may keep the mind too alert to fall asleep.

- Depression. This is a very pronounced reason to keep people alert and make sleep difficult.
- Long-term use of sleep medication. Drugs such as Ambian or Wellbutrian cause psychological dependence on them.
- Pain. Many conditions, including arthritis, fibromyalgia, neuropathy, trigeminal neuralgia, plus assorted injuries, will cause pain, making it hard to fall asleep and stay asleep.
- Aging. When people age, they do not need as much sleep as they did when young. The reasons for this include changing life patterns, family changes, and other worries, all of which can cause insomnia.

TREATMENTS IN WESTERN MEDICINE

From the perspective of Western medicine, there are two major types of treatments.

Non-Medicinal Treatments and Behavioral Therapy

- Sleep hygiene. This is a component of behavioral therapy, with several simple steps that can be taken to improve the quality and quantity of sleep, such as timing of sleep, food intake, sleeping environment etc. Sleep hygiene combines advice about aspects of sleep control, how to avoid sleep deprivation, and how to respond to unwanted sleep interruptions if they occur.

- Increased exercise. Exercising a minimum of 45 minutes a day, 6 days a week, will greatly improve the quality of sleep.
- Relaxation therapy. Massage, meditation, muscle relaxation, or a hot bath or shower can assist in falling, and staying, asleep. No one should ever try to force themselves to sleep, but should retire in a relaxed mood.
- It is best to keep a regular sleeping and waking schedule and not drink caffeine, or any beverage, before sleeping. Nor is it good to smoke. Do not go to bed hungry, and make sure the sleeping chamber is adjusted for light, temperature, and noise to make sleeping easier.
- Stimulus control: It's important to go to bed as soon as you feel sleepy, and not watch television, read, eat, or worry in bed. It is not advisable to take long naps during the day. (Oversleeping does not improve insomnia.)

Medication

- Benzodiazepines. There are many different types, including temazepam, lorazepam, triazolam, and clonazepam. All of these benzodiazepines are very effective in improving the quality and quantity of sleep.
- Nonbenzodiazepine medicine, which includes Lunesta, Sonata, and Ambien.
- Melatonin. This is a hormone secreted by the pineal gland. It is produced during the night and helps

body relaxation. (Attention needed here, however, because regular use causes the body to permanently lose its ability to produce the hormone.)

- Rozeren. This will stimulate the melatonin receptor to improve sleep quality and quantity.
- Some antidepressants, such as Elavil, Endep, or Desyrel, have also been used for a long time to aid in depression as well as sleep.
- Antihistamines. Benadryl, for example, and other antihistamines can be used to induce drowsiness. The drawback to this is that, during the day, they can make it dangerous for a patient to drive or operate machinery.

TREATMENTS IN TRADITIONAL CHINESE MEDICINE

Chinese medicine indicates five types of insomnia.

Excessive Fire in the Heart and Liver

The main symptom is irritability, difficulty falling asleep, sleeping intermittently, waking up easily, sometimes experiencing dizziness, dry mouth, bitter taste in the mouth, and dry tongue body, with yellowish coating on the tongue and a rapid pulse. The method of treatment is to decrease the excessive fire of the liver and heart. The acupuncture points are Liver 2 Xing Jian, GB

20 Feng Chi, Heart 7 Sheng Men, ExHN 13 An Mian.

TABLE 23.1

POINTS	MERIDIAN NUMBER	CONDITIONS HELPED
1 Xing Jian	Liver 2. See Figure 23.1	Insomnia, abdominal distension, headaches, dizziness and vertigo, congestion, swelling and eye pain, deviation of the mouth, hernia, painful urination, retention of urine, irregular menstruation, epilepsy, convulsions
2 Feng Chi	GB 20. See Figure 12.1	See Table 12.1
3 Sheng Men	Heart 7. See Figure 20.2	See Table 20.2
4 An Mian	Ex HN13. See Figure 23.2	Insomnia, vertigo, headaches, palpitations, mental disorders

Please refer to the accompanying Figures (illustrations) for the locations of the points. And please note that these illustrations are for information only and may not show all the exact locations of the acupuncture points.

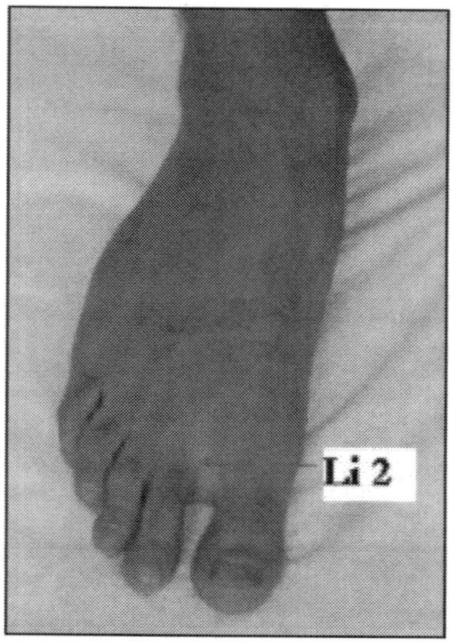

FIGURE 23.1

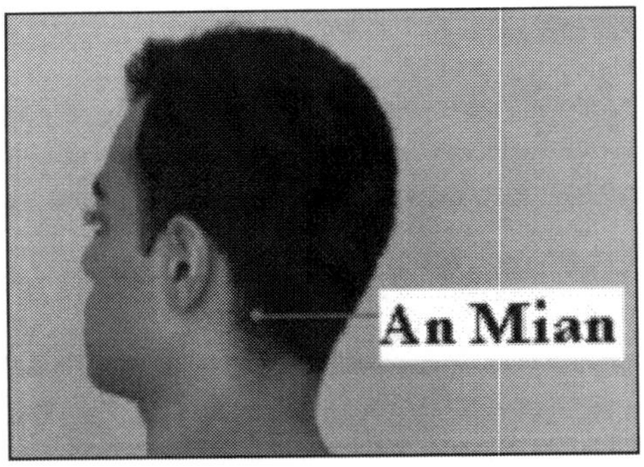

FIGURE 23.2

These points can calm the mind and improve sleep. Xing Jian belongs to the liver meridian which, when treated, can decrease the fire of the heart and liver. Feng Chi is located in the gallbladder meridian, and together with Sheng Men, a point of the heart meridian, they will decrease the fire of the liver and heart, and help to calm the brain. An Mian is also a very important point for alleviating insomnia.

Overeating

Many people experience a restless night after overeating; they feel bloated and gaseous, and have constipation or diarrhea, with white coating on the tongue. The treatment is to strengthen the spleen and stomach to calm the mind and induce sleep. The acupuncture points are Pi Shu, Zu San Li, Sheng Men, and An Mian. Pi Shu and Zu San Li are the best points for the stomach bloating, constipation, and diarrhea. Digestion will be much improved by stimulating Pi Shu and Zu San Li. As mentioned, Sheng Men and An Mian will greatly facilitate sleep.

TABLE 23.2

POINTS	MERIDIAN NUMBER	CONDITIONS HELPED
1 Pi Shu	UB 20. See Figure 18.3	See Table 18.1
2 Zu San Li	Stomach 36. See Figure 13.4	See Table 13.3
3 Sheng Men	Heart 7. See Figure 20.2	See Table 20.2
4 An Mian	Ex HN13. See Figure 23.2	Insomnia, Vertigo

Please refer to the accompanying Figures (illustrations) for the locations of the points. And please note that these illustrations are for information only and may not show all the exact locations of the acupuncture points.

Depression and Sadness with Deficiency of Lung Energy

The main symptoms are depression, low energy, slowed conversation with low tone, accompanied by congested lungs, difficulty sleeping, and always waking up during the night. Sometimes there is a shortness of breath and a thin white coating on the tongue, with a deeply weak pulse. The points should be Fei Shu, Lie Que, Sheng Men, and An Mian. The acupuncture points will help the energy of spleen, stomach, and lung to improve their function.

TABLE 23.3

POINTS	MERIDIAN NUMBER	CONDITIONS HELPED
1 Fei Shu	UB 13. See Figure 13.1	See Table 13.1
2 Lie Que	Lung 7. See Figure 12.2	See Table 12.1

POINTS	MERIDIAN NUMBER	CONDITIONS HELPED
3 Sheng Men	Heart 7. See Figure 20.2	See Table 20.2
4 An Mian	Ex HN 13. See figure 23.2	Insomnia, vertigo, headaches, palpitations, mental disorders

Please refer to the accompanying Figures (illustrations) for the locations of the points. And please note that these illustrations are for information only and may not show all the exact locations of the acupuncture points.

Disharmony of the Heart and Kidney

The main symptoms are anxiety, chest pain, difficulty maintaining asleep and easily waking up, heart palpitations, and stress, as well as weakness of the low back and legs, night sweats, and hot flashes, with red coating of the tongue and rapid and weak pulse. The points are Sheng Shu, Tai Xi, Sheng Men, and An Main.

TABLE 23.4

POINTS	MERIDIAN NUMBER	CONDITIONS HELPED
1 Sheng Shu	UB 23. See Figure 14.1	See Table 14.4
2 Tai Xi	Kidney 3. See Figure 16.6	See Table 16.2
3 Sheng Men	Heart 7. See Figure 20.2	See Table 20.2
4 An Mian	Ex HN 13. See Fig-ure 23.2	Insomnia, vertigo, headaches, palpitations, mental disorders

Please refer to the accompanying Figures (illustrations) for the locations of the points. And please note that these illustrations are for information only and may not show all the exact locations of the acupuncture points.

Deficiency of Qi (Energy) and Blood

The main symptoms of this type of insomnia are dizziness, drowsiness, forgetfulness, poor sleep, tinnitus, and weakness, as well as cold in all the extremities, a pale face and tongue, poor digestion, and a weak pulse. The method of treatment is to calm the mind, and tonify the blood and qi, thus improving sleep. The points are Pi Shu, Sheng Shu, San Yin Jiao, Sheng Men, and An Mian.

TABLE 23.5

POINTS	MERIDIAN NUMBER	CONDITIONS HELPED
1 Pi Shu	UB 20. See Figure 18.3	See Table 18.1
2 Sheng Shu	UB 23. See Figure 14.1	See Table 14.4
3 San Yin Jiao	Spleen 6. See Figure 16.7	See Table 16.1
3 Sheng Men	Heart 7. See Figure 20.2	See Table 20.2
4 An Mian	Ex HN13. See Figure 23.2	Insomnia, vertigo, headaches, palpitations, mental disorders

Please refer to the accompanying Figures (illustrations) for the locations of the points. And please note that these illustrations are for information only and may not show all the exact locations of the acupuncture points.

ALICE'S TREATMENT

Since stress caused her poor sleep, Alice belongs to type three. I selected the acupuncture points UB 13 Fei Shu, Lu 7 Lie Que, Heart 7 Sheng Men, and Ex HNI3 An Mian, and she reported that, after the first treatment, she slept three to four hours. After the second week, her sleeping increased to five or six hours a night and she was starting to feel much better. Ater a month, her sleep pattern became normal, and she could sleep through the night. Her husband's news that he found a job locally and would no longer have to commute to New York also alleviated her stress, which further helped her establish a normal pattern of sleep. Ater her course of treatment, Alice thanked me for how much I had helped her achieve relief from her insomnia.

TIPS FOR PERSONAL USE AT HOME

- Take a hot shower and then press An Mian points (see Figure 23.2) for 15 minutes on each side before you go to bed. Acupressure the points with your thumb or knuckle, pressing with comfortable pressure on the points.
- Do not force yourself go to bed if you do not have desire to sleep.
- Do physical exercise at least 45 minutes per day, 6 days per week. The exercise will help you a lot.

24

Tinnitus

RINGING IN JOHN'S EAR

John, a sixty-seven-year-old man, recently retired from teaching high school, then went back to work as a security guard at the school gate. Whenever he begins to read, he starts to experience sound within his ear, though there is no corresponding external sound. The off-and-on sound can be a strong ringing noise in his right ear, a high-pitched whining noise, buzzing, or hissing. If he pays attention to something else, he does not experience the tinnitus, but if he is idle or preparing to go to sleep, the sound recurs and can interfere with his ability to either concentrate or hear, which is very frustrating. He consulted several doctors, including an ENT specialist and a neurologist. The ENT doctor checked his outer, middle, and inner ears, and found no infection or allergies, and no edema in the ear. The neurologist ordered a CT scan and an MRI, which did not show a tumor or any problem with the brain. He was prescribed such medications as Xanax and tricyclic antidepressants, as well as niacin, all to no avail. At this point he was referred to me for evaluation.

I determined that John probably had tinnitus, the symptoms of which are hearing phantom sounds in the ear, including buzzing, clicking, hissing, ringing, or whistling, when there is no external noise. The sounds may vary in pitch from a low roar to a high squeal, and the person may hear it in one or both ears. The sound is sometimes continuous, sometimes intermittent, and it may interfere with the ability to concentrate. When the person is nervous or experiences stress, the tinnitus becomes worse.

TYPES OF TINNITUS

There are two types of tinnitus.

1. Subjective tinnitus is the most common form, and only the person can hear or feel it in this type. About one fifth of the population complains of this kind of tinnitus, which can be caused by ear problems in the outer, middle, or inner ear. It can also be caused by problems with the auditory nerves or the brain stem, which can interrupt the nerve signals as sound.
2. Objective tinnitus is the type where both the patient and the doctor doing the examination can feel the sound. This is the rare type of the condition. It can be a muscular issue, or it can be caused by blood vessel or inner-ear bone problems.

CAUSES OF TINNITUS

There are many causes of tinnitus, but the most common is hearing loss. As people age, they lose hearing because of tremors to the ear through noise, drugs, or chemicals, which damage the portion of the ear that allows them to hear. Examples include acoustic shock, external ear infection, ear-wax impaction, lead or mercury poisoning, Menière's disease, or such toxic medications as aspirin, erythromycin, or tetracycline. There are also neurological disorders, such as head injuries, psychiatric disorders, such as depression and anxiety, sclerosis, or metabolic disorders, such as thyroid problems, hyperlipidemia, and vitamin B_{12} deficiency.

TREATMENTS IN WESTERN MEDICINE

Objective Tinnitus

For this type of tinnitus, the obvious cause needs to be treated. If there is an acoustic tumor or an infection, the tumor should be removed, or the infection alleviated. These might make the tinnitus disappear or decrease in intensity. While there are many different treatments for tinnitus, none has proven to be entirely reliable. Western medicine treats this condition with gamma knife radiosurgery, cochlear implants, Botox, or medications, such as propanol and clonazepam.

Subjective Tinnitus

For this type of tinnitus, the treatment might be lidocaine injections to the inner ear, and benzodiazepine to calm the person and decrease his or her anxiety, tricyclic antidepressants to decrease depression, or carbamazepine and melatonin to help decrease the tinnitus. None of these treatments show any statistical difference in the cure of tinnitus. Other methods include electrical stimulation, such as transcranial direct current stimulation, or direct stimulation to the auditory cortex by implanting electrodes.

TREATMENTS IN TRADITIONAL CHINESE MEDICINE

Traditional Chinese medicine believes there are two main causes for tinnitus.

- Excessive fire attack is one cause. The gallbladder meridians go up to the top of the head and around the ear; if there is excessive heat, this will go through the ear and cause blockage of energy, so the meridians cannot transmit normal sound to the inner ear. This type of tinnitus is high pitched, usually accompanied by anxiety, headaches, and sometimes fear, dry mouth, constipation, yellowish urine, and red face; sometimes the chest feels uncomfortable and painful, with red tongue body and yellow tongue coating. The treatments mostly used are SJ 5 Wai Guan, SJ 17 Yi Feng, SI 19 Ting Gong, SJ 21 Er Meng, UB 18 Gan Shu, and Liv 3 Tai Chong.
- Yin deficiency syndrome. The person feels weak and has a pale face, and the tinnitus is slow and

low in pitch; sometimes it is off and on, with the pitch sound decreasing when the person holds her or his breath. This form of tinnitus is often accompanied by dizziness, faintness, shortness of breath, tiredness, and weakness of the legs; sometimes there is a low-grade fever, the palms are hot, there is no taste in the mouth, with a very thin coating on the tongue and a weak pulse. This type belongs to a yin deficiency and the treatment should be to tonify the yin and enhance the kidney. The acupuncture points are UB 23 Sheng Shu, Kid 4 Tai Xi, SJ 17 Yi Feng, SJ 21 Er Meng, SI 19 Ting Gong, GB 2 Ting Hui, SJ 5 Wai Guan, and UB 18 Gan Shu. (See Table 24.1 below for the location of these points.)

TABLE 24.1

POINTS	MERIDIAN NUMBER	CONDITIONS HELPED
1 Wai Guan	SJ S. See Figure 1 2.3	See Table 12.2
2 Y Feng	SJ 17. See Figure 25.1	See Table 25.1
3 Ting Gong	SI 19. See Figure 25.1	See Table 25.1
4 Er Meng	Si 21. See Figure 25.1	See Table 25.1
5 Gan Shu	UB 18. See Figure 19.1	See Table 19.1
6 Sheng Shu	UB23. See Figure 14.1	See Table 14.4
7 Tai Chong	Liv 3. See Figure 18.2	See Table 18.1
8 Tai Xi	Kid 4. See Figure 16.7	See Table 16.2
9 Ting Hui	GB 2. See Figure 25.1	See Table 25.2

Please refer to the accompanying Figures (illustrations) for the locations of the points. And please note that these illustrations are for information only and may not show all the exact locations of the acupuncture points.

JOHN'S TREATMENT

John underwent TCM treatment for excessive heat with SI 19 Ting Gong and GB 2 Ting Hui points on both sides, and Liv 3 Tai Chong and St 36 Zu San Li, all of which were utilized to decrease excessive heat in the kidney and to improve his kidney and stomach function. After one month, John reported that he began to experience a decrease in the pitch of the tinnitus, and after two months, he reported that he heard no sounds about 70 percent of the time. He was advised to do some exercises and learn to deal with stress, and after three months of treatment his condition was much improved.

In my personal experience, the Ting Gong, Ting Hui, and Er Meng are the most important points, and by using this acupuncture treatment plus electrical stimulation each session for 30 minutes three times a week for a month, the tinnitus symptoms will most likely greatly decrease.

TIPS FOR PERSONAL USE AT HOME OR OFFICE

- Always massage points SJ 21, SI 19, and GB 2 for 30 minutes each session, 2 sessions per day. Acupressure the points with your thumb or knuckle, pressing with comfortable pressure on the points. You should work symmetric points at the same time.

- Try to avoid loud sounds.

25

Hearing Loss

LISA'S HEARING LOSS

Lisa is a fifty-four-year-old woman who came to me complaining that she had started experiencing hearing loss six months before. At that time, for no apparent reason, she'd had a sudden onset of Bell's palsy on the left side of her face. That side of her face drooped, she had difficulty drinking water, and she had trouble closing her left eye. The doctor who diagnosed her condition told her she might recover spontaneously in a few months, and advised her to massage the left side of her face on a daily basis. She followed his advice and, fortunately, recovered from Bell's palsy, but shortly thereafter started to lose hearing in her left ear. She noticed a muffled quality to speech and other sounds that made it difficult to understand words, especially in crowded situations or noisy backgrounds, and she had to ask people to speak more clearly and loudly, an embarrassment at her age. Lisa began to feel withdrawn from conversations and started avoiding social situations where she had to turn her head toward the speaker in order to hear better. Frustrated, she came to me for evaluation.

THE THREE TYPES OF HEARING LOSS

Hearing loss can be categorized by where or what part of the auditory system is damaged. There are three basic types of hearing loss: Conductive hearing loss, sensorineural hearing loss, and mixed hearing loss.

Conductive Hearing Loss of the External or Middle Ear

This hearing loss is involved in the conductive pathway of the external and middle ear. It occurs when sound is not efficiently conducted through the outer ear canal to the eardrum and the tiny bones, or ossicles, of the middle ear. Conductive hearing loss usually involves a reduction in sound level, or a reduced ability to hear faint sounds. This type of hearing loss can often be medically or surgically corrected.

- **External Ear.** In this type, a partial or complete occlusion of the ear canal by ear wax is a frequent cause of conductive hearing loss. Warm water irrigation or the use of an otoscope and a curette allows the wax to be removed under direct vision. Please do not use a Q-tip, as this will occlude the external canal more.

Reasons for this type of problem include foreign bodies, an infection of the skin of the external auditory canal, and benign bony growths of the external auditory canal that interfere with normal wax migration, leading to occlusion and conductive hearing loss.

- **Middle Ear.** Middle ear pathology may lead to conductive hearing loss, including such problems as fluid in the middle ear from colds, allergies, serious otitis media, poor function of the eustachian tube, ear infection, perforated eardrum, and benign tumors.

Sensorineural Hearing Loss of the Inner Ear

Sensorineural hearing loss encompasses disorders that affect the inner ear when there is damage to it or to the nerve pathways from the inner ear to the brain. Sensorineural hearing loss cannot be medically or surgically corrected. Sensorineural hearing loss not only involves a reduction in sound level or ability to hear faint sounds, but also affects speech understanding or the ability to hear clearly. Sensorineural hearing loss can be caused by drugs that are toxic to the auditory system, genetic syndromes and diseases, such as Bell's palsy or meningitis, and birth injuries. A hearing-test screen is required for all newborn babies because hearing loss can cause a delay in their development. Other causes of this type of hearing loss include a noisy environment, viruses, head trauma, aging, and tumors.

Mixed Conductive and Sensorineural Hearing Loss

Sometimes a conductive hearing loss occurs in combination with a sensorineural hearing loss. This type of loss includes injury to the outer or middle ear, as well as to the auditory nerve in the inner ear. When this occurs, the hearing loss is referred to as a mixed hearing loss.

For further information, see the website for the American Speech-Language-Hearing Association: www.asha.org/public/hearing/disorders/types.htm

TREATMENTS IN WESTERN MEDICINE

- For conductive hearing loss, the first step is to treat the cause of the loss. With ear infections, use antibiotics. If there is fluid block in the middle ear, drain the fluid; if the ear is impacted with ear wax, clean it out; or, if there is a foreign body, pick it out.
- For sensorineural hearing loss, Western medicine has no really good treatment, and doctors typically prescribe hearing aids. They treat this type of loss as permanent and believe there is no relief. If the loss is severe, owing to damage in the inner ear, an electronic device called a cochlear implant may be used, which connects the inner-ear nerve

to the brain to help the person recover from nerve damage.

TREATMENTS IN TRADITIONAL CHINESE MEDICINE

TCM believes sensorineural hearing loss is due to energy blockage in the gallbladder meridian because this meridian surrounds the ear and sends energy to the brain. If this blockage occurs, then the nerve cannot function normally and the hearing will be injured.

There are two major types of hearing loss based on concepts in traditional Chinese medicine.

Excessive Pattern

TABLE 25.1

POINTS	MERIDIAN NUMBER	CONDITIONS HELPED
1 Wai Guan	Si 5. See Figure 12.3	See Table 12.2
2 Y Feng	Si 17. See Figure 25.1	7. See Figure 25.1 Deafness, facial paralysis, swelling of the cheek, tinnitus, toothache
3 Er Meng	Si 21. See Figure 25.1	Deafness, stiffness of the lip, tinnitus, toothache
4 Gan Shu	UB 18. See Figure 19.1	See Table 19.3
5 Tai Chong	Liver 3. See Figure 18.2	See Table 18.1

POINTS	MERIDIAN NUMBER	CONDITIONS HELPED
6 Xia Xi	GB 43. See Figure 25.2	Deafness, dizziness, headaches, swelling of the cheek, tinnitus, vertigo

Please refer to the accompanying Figures (illustrations) for the locations of the points. And please note that these illustrations are for information only and may not show all the exact locations of the acupuncture points.

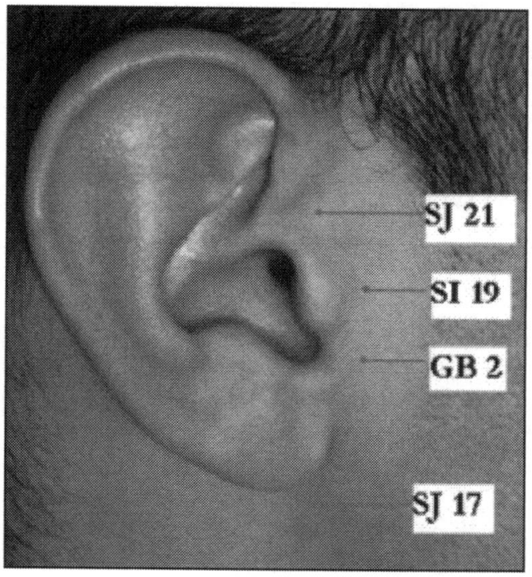

FIGURE 25.1

With this hearing decrease or loss, the person usually has a strong body structure and gets easily excited. He or she has high-pitch tinnitus, headaches, slightly increased body temperature, dry and bitter mouth, constipation and yellowish urine, reddish face, chest tightness, and an uncomfortable, red tongue body with yellowish coating on the tongue.

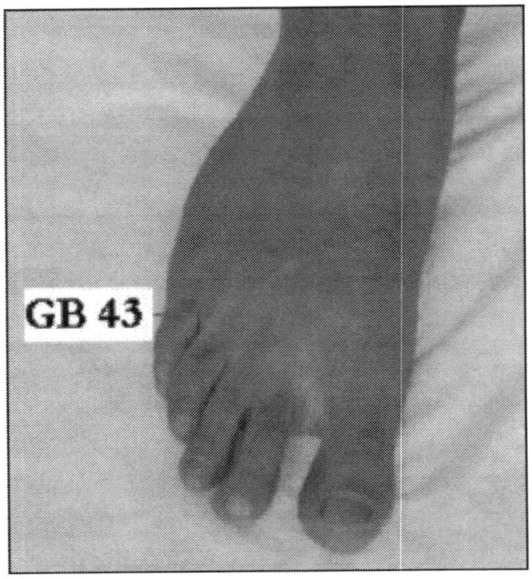

FIGURE 25.2

The acupuncture points for this pattern of diminished hearing are Wai Guan, Yi Feng, Ting Gong, Er Meng, Gan Shu, Tai Chong, and Xia Xi.

Deficiency Pattern

The person with this hearing decrease or loss is usually thin and has a weak body structure. She or he has a whitish face, a low, mild, or trace-pitch sound in the ear, tiredness and fatigue, dizziness, weakness in the legs, night sweats, (sometimes) hot flashes, no taste in the mouth, and a pale tongue body with thin coating.

The acupuncture points for this pattern of diminished hearing are Sheng Shu, Tai Xi, Yi Feng, Er Meng, Ting Gong, Ting Hui, Wai Guan, and Gan Shu.

TABLE 25.2

POINTS	MERIDIAN NUMBER	CONDITIONS HELPED
1 Sheng Shu	UB 23. See Figure 14.1	See Table 14.4
2 Tai Xi	Kidney 3. See Figure 15.7	See Table 16.2
3 Y Feng	SJ 17. See Figure 25.1	See Figure 25.1
4 Er Meng	SJ 21. See Figure 25.1	See Figure 25.1
5 Ting Gong	SI 19. See Figure 25.1	Deafness, motor impairment of the mandibular (jaw) joint, tinnitus, toothache
6 Ting Hui	GB 2. See Figure 25.1	Deafness, deviation of the eye and mouth, motor impairment of the mandibular (jaw) joint, mumps, tinnitus, toothache
7 Wai Guan	SJ 5. See Figure 12.3	See Table 12.2
8 Gan Shu	UB 18. See Figure 19.1	See Table 19.3

Please refer to the accompanying Figures (illustrations) for the locations of the points. And please note that these illustrations are for information only and may not show all the exact locations of the acupuncture points.

LISA'S TREATMENT

Lisa was treated three times a week for six weeks, after which she reported that her hearing had improved and she no longer needed to turn her head toward the origin of conversations. She no longer experiences a muffled quality of speech when people converse with her and is more and more active, enjoying social situations as she once had.

TIPS TO USE AT HOME OR OFFICE

- The earlier you seek acupuncture treatment, the better result you will get.
- Acupuncture cannot treat every hearing loss disease. If your middle ear nerve is severely damaged, it may not help.
- Massaging acupressure points SJ 21, SI 19, GB 2, and SJ 17 for 5 minutes per point, 2 sessions per day, will greatly help with your hearing. Acupressure with your thumb or knuckle, pressing with comfortable pressure on the points. You should work symmetric points at the same time.

26

Strokes

WILLIAM'S STROKE

William H., a seventy-year-old man with a history of hypertension and diabetes mellitus, came to my office complaining that his left arm and leg had been weak and almost paralyzed for two months. He told me that several months earlier he had experienced a sudden-onset headache. He had felt numbness and a tingling sensation in his left arm and leg, had difficulty opening both eyes, experienced double vision as well as slurred speech and dizziness, and his movements were clumsy. He was rushed to the emergency room where he was given a CT scan, which confirmed that he'd had a stroke. He was immediately admitted to the hospital and was given all possible medical treatment: anticoagulation medication, aspirin, and heparin. He remained in the hospital for a month and, upon discharge, he entered an acute rehab center where he was given exercises for his arm and leg. After a month he felt some improvement in his shoulder and hip joints, but still could not move his elbow, wrist, fingers, knee, or ankles. Finally, he consulted me for treatment.

TYPES AND CAUSES OF STROKES

Strokes usually occur in down time, and are usually heralded by all or some of these symptoms: a sudden onset of weakness or paralysis of the arms, legs, side of the face, or any part of the body. They can be accompanied by numbness and a decreased tingling sensation, with slurred speech, an inability to speak or understand someone's else speech, difficulty reading or writing, blurred vision, difficulty swallowing, drooling, loss of balance or coordination, loss of memory, and vertigo. Some people also experience anxiety, depression, lethargy, nervous energy, or loss of consciousness. These symptoms are usually caused by a blockage in the brain artery, a narrowing of the small arteries within the brain, or a hardening of the arteries and arthrosclerosis leading to the brain.

Strokes are usually divided into three types.

- Type 1 is ischemic stroke, caused by a blood clot that blocks blood flow to the brain.
- Type 2 is hemorrhagic stroke, caused by bleeding inside of the brain that is secondary to ruptured aneurysms or uncontrolled high blood pressure.
- Type 3 is a transient ischemic attack (TIA). This symptom is seen for less than twenty-four hours, after which the person recovers and becomes normal again. A TIA is a warning stroke, or mini-stroke that produces strokelike symptoms, but no lasting damage. Recognizing and treating TIAs can reduce your risk of a major stroke.

Additional causes of strokes, with the exception of strokes caused by old age or high blood pressure, are described below.

- Coronary artery disease, which can lead to a heart attack or stroke, as can other heart conditions, such as endocarditis, fibrillation, heart failure, or heart valve diseases.
- Diabetes, which doubles the risk of stroke.
- High cholesterol, which causes hardening of the arteries.
- Overweight and diet. Consumption of high-fat food and alcohol abuse can cause a stroke. Too much alcohol increases blood pressure and cholesterol levels.
- Peripheral artery disease, such as carotid artery disease.
- Physical inactivity.
- Smoking, both primary and secondhand.

TREATMENTS IN WESTERN MEDICINE

In Western medicine, strokes are treated as follows.

Ischemic Strokes

- In an ischemic stroke the doctor must quickly restore blood flow to the brain. This emergency treatment, together with medication, usually starts with aspirin, which has proved the best treatment immediately after a stroke, and reduces the possibility of another stroke. The emergency room doctor will likely administer this treatment.

- Two other useful drugs for treating ischemic strokes are coumadin and heparin.
- Some who have ischemic strokes may be given tissue plasminogen activator (rt-PA), which is a potent clot-busting drug that helps some people fully recover. According to recent N.I.H. protocol, rt-PA must be injected within 3 hours after the symptoms' onset, once brain bleeding is ruled out by CT scan and/or doctors are certain that giving a tissue plasminogen activator (TPA) will not worsen any bleeding in the brain. TPA is administered only in ischemic strokes.
- Surgical procedures might also be used, including carotid endarterectomy, angioplasty, and stents.

Hemorrhagic Strokes Where Surgery Must be Utilized

The most common procedures for hemorrhagic strokes are clipping aneurysms and removal of an arteriovenous malformation (AVM). This is an abnormal connection between veins and arteries, usually congenital, and usually occurring in the central nervous system.

After emergency treatment, early rehabilitation is very important because the most benefit will be obtained within six months of having a stroke.

There will usually be a team of doctors and therapists to help with stroke recovery. It can consist of a dietician, a neurophysiologist, a nurse, occupational, physical, and recreational therapists, a psychiatrist, a rehabilitation doctor, a social worker, and a speech therapist. The goal of stroke rehabilitation is to help the person recover as much independence and function as possible. Much of stroke rehabilitation involves relearning the skills of daily activity, not only for the paralyzed extremities, but also for improving speech and swallowing, as well as for vision and hearing functions.

TREATMENTS IN TRADITIONAL CHINESE MEDICINE

The TCM treatments for strokes are different from Western medicine, where, after emergency room treatment or surgery, the main recovery method is to try and return physical functions to the parts of the body affected by the stroke. Although this method will strengthen the muscles and increase the range of motion, the goal of TCM and acupuncture is to try and stimulate the seat of the stroke, the brain—a method that is believed to help the patient recover more quickly.

Both Western and traditional Chinese medicine recognize the same two forms of stroke: Ischemic and hemorrhagic. Acupuncture should be started as soon as possible after a stroke occurs and the person's medical condition has been stabilized.

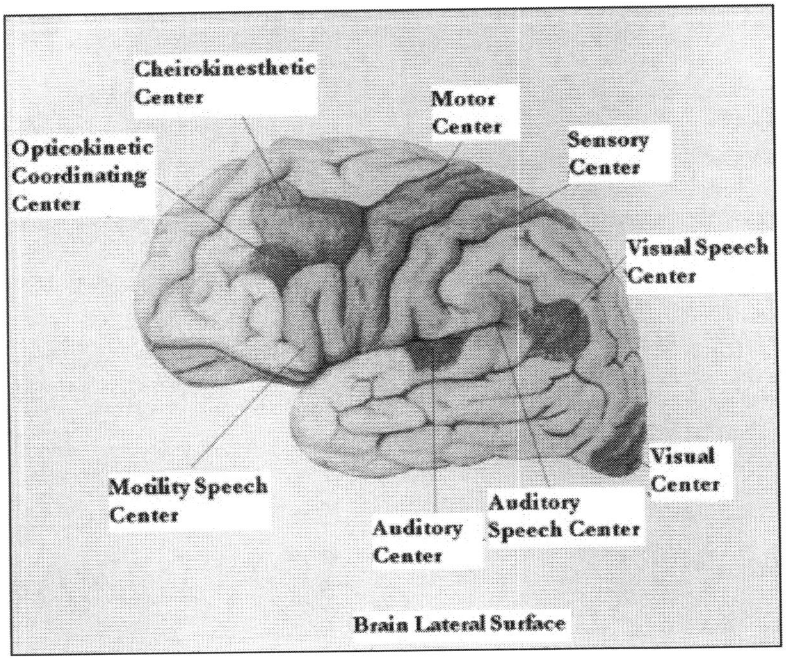

FIGURE 26.1A

As illustrated in Figure 26.1A, the brain contains many different functional centers. On the motor and sensory zones, as shown in Figure 26.1B, the brain structure looks like an upside down human body, functionally represented on the cerebral cortex.

EXPLANATION OF POINTS

- Cheirokinesthetic Center: Center for memories of movements

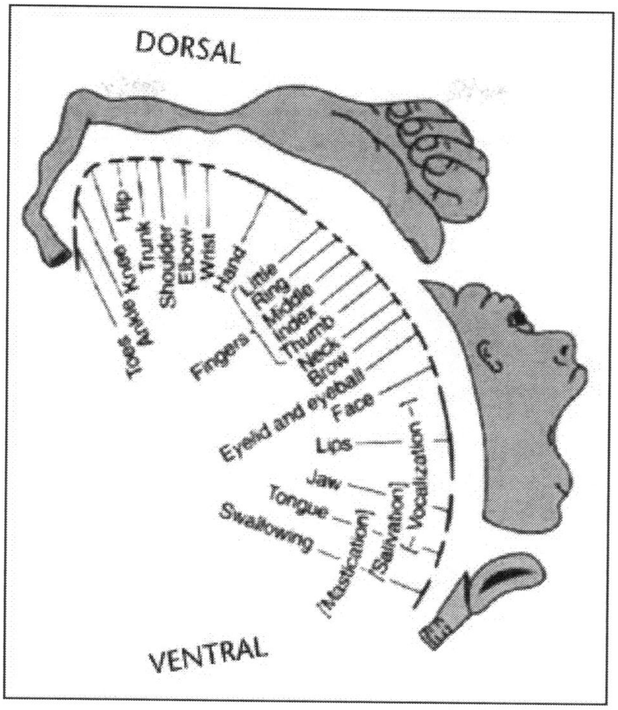

FIGURE 26.1B

- Opticokinetic Coordinating Center: Center for movement of the eyeballs in response to the movement of objects across the visual field
- Motility Speech Center: Center for movements related to speech organs
- Auditory Center: Center for primary processing of hearing; center for receiving impulses from the ear by way of the auditory nerve
- Auditory Speech Center: Center for interpretation of sound
- Visual Center: Center for receiving signal from eyes.
- Visual Speech Center: Center for understanding of the written and spoken language; enables a

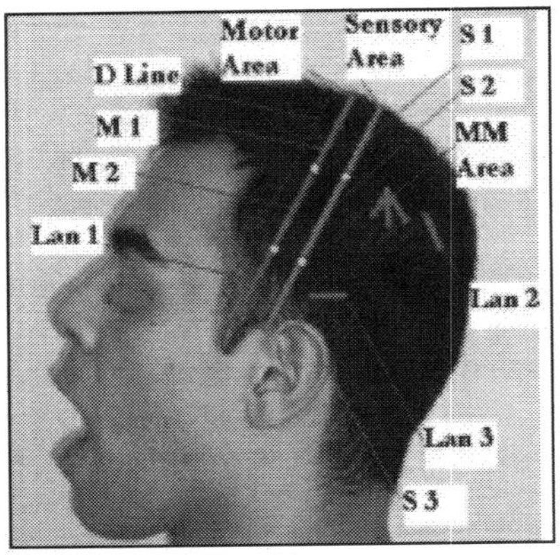

FIGURE 26.2

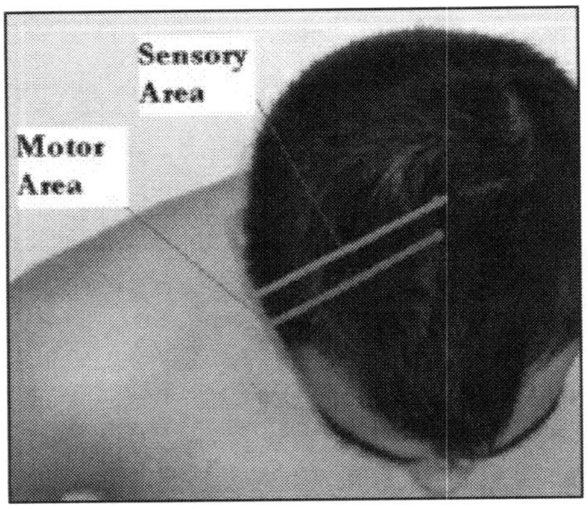

FIGURE 26.3

person to read a sentence, understand it and say it out loud

- Sensory Center: Center for entire body's sensation
- Motor Center: Center for entire body's movement

Figure 26.1B illustrates the location of movement of the body's entire trunk and four limbs. Please refer to its motor area in Figure 26.1A.

During the course of more than three thousand years of accumulated experience, traditional Chinese medicine (TCM) developed scalp acupuncture, one of its most advanced treatments for people with strokes.

TCM studied the relationship between the human body's function and the anatomy of the scalp, and created systemic points on the scalp, which coincide with contemporary neuroanatomy.

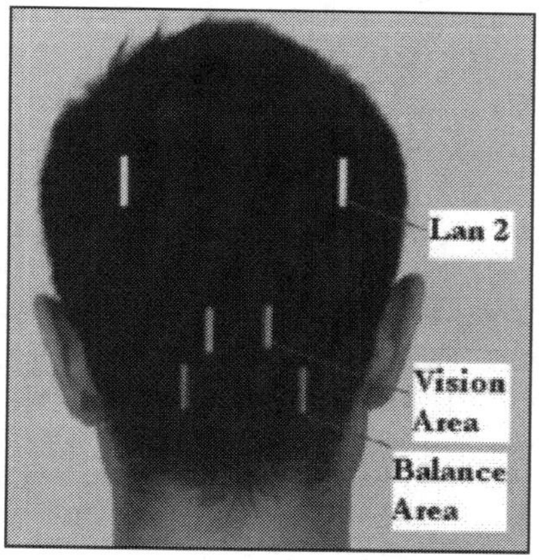

FIGURE 26.4

The Importance of Acupuncture Treatments

The most valuable treatment of TCM for strokes is the combination of body and scalp acupuncture. The cause of a stroke is the occluded blood supply to the brain, but the focus of current rehab medicine is mainly on the upper and lower extremities—hundreds of hours are spent on rehabilitation for these upper and lower extremities. Most physical and occupational therapies are designed for both sets of extremities, but there is no exercise or treatment designed for the brain. With acupuncture, however, not only are these extremities treated, but the *cause* of the stroke is treated as well with the use of body and scalp acupuncture. It is important to change the medical concepts about stroke rehabilitation because the problem is the *brain* and doctors not only need to work on the body, but also on the brain.

Acupuncture Treatments for TIAs—Transient Ischemic Attacks

In TIAs, there is dizziness, weakness on one side of the body, with numbness and a tingling sensation, and the symptoms gradually disappear within twenty-four hours. The following points are used with TIAs.

- Body points: Du 23 Shang Xin, Du 20 Bai Hui, Ex-HN 3 Ying Tang, LI 15 Jian Yu, LI 11 Qu Qi, St 36 Zu San Li, and GB 34 Yang Ling Quan.
- Scalp points: Motor and Sensory area. (Figure 26.3)

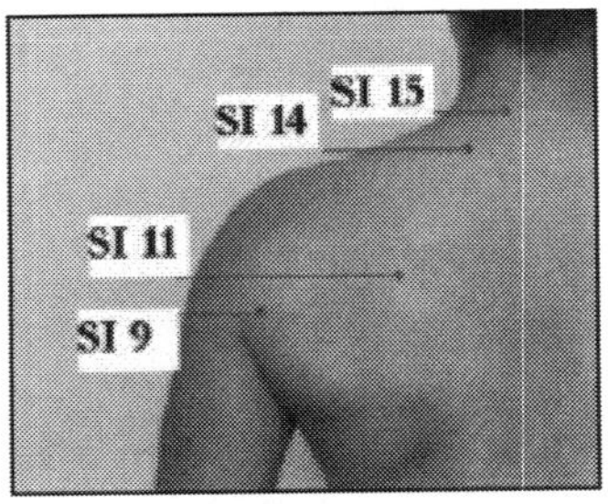

FIGURE 26.5

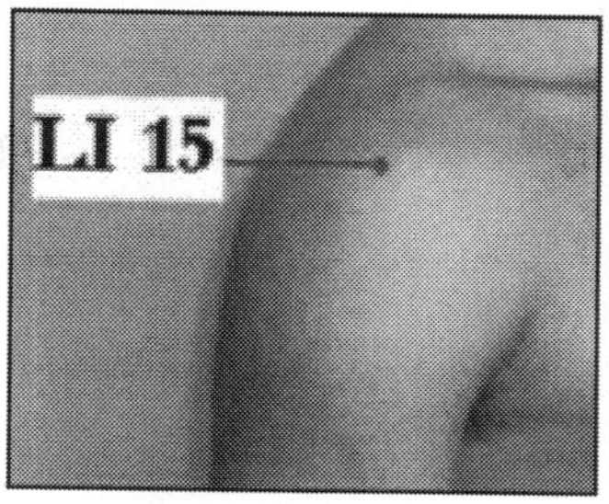

FIGURE 26.6

TABLE 26.1

POINTS	MERIDIAN NUMBER	CONDITIONS HELPED
1 Shang Xin	Du 23. See Figure 29.3	Headaches, eye pain, running nose, mental disorders
2 Bai Hui	Du 20. See Figure 16.4	See Table 16.2
3 Ying Tang	Ex–HN 3. See Figure 22.1	See Table 22.1
4 Jian Yu	LI 15. See Figure 26.6	Shoulder and arm pain, motor impairment of the upper extremities, rubella, skin disease
5 Qu Qi	LI 11. See Figure 12.2	See Table 12.2
6 Zu San Li	St 36. See Figure 13.4	See Table 13.
7 Yang Ling Quan	GB 34. See Figure 15.3	See Table 15.3

Please refer to the accompanying Figures (illustrations) for the locations of the points. And please note that these illustrations are for information only and may not show all the exact locations of the acupuncture points.

Acupuncture Treatments for Ischemic Strokes

Symptoms of ischemic strokes are facial paralysis, sluggish language, and paralysis on one side of the body. The following points are used with ischemic strokes.

- Body points: PC 6 Nei Guan, Du 26 Ren Zhong, Sp 6 San Yin Jiao, Ht 1 Ji quan, Lu 5 Qi Zhe, UB 40 Wei Zhong, LI 4 He Gu, and LI 11 Qu Qi.
- Scalp points: Motor and Sensory area, especially, M1, M2, S3, Lan 1, Lan 2, and Lan 3.

TABLE 26.2

POINTS	MERIDIAN NUMBER	CONDITIONS HELPED
1 Nei Guan	PC 6. See Figure 16.7	See Table 16.1
2 Ren Zhong	Du 26. See Figure 29.3	Mental disorders, seizure, hysteria, infantile convulsion, coma, apoplexy, off–center deviation of the mouth and eyes, puffiness of the face, low back pain, and stiffness
3 San Ying Jiao	Sp 6. See Figure 16.6	See Table 16.1
4 Ji Quan	Heart 1. See Figure 26.7	Pain in the rib and cardiac regions, scrofula (skin disease), cold pain of elbow and arm, dry throat
5 Qi Zhe	Lu 5. See Figure 13.2	See Table 13.2
6 Wei Zhong	UB 40. See Figure 26.8	Low back pain, motor impairment of the hip joint, muscular atrophy, pain, numbness, and motor impairment of the legs, abdominal pain, vomiting, diarrhea
7 He Gu	LI 4. See Figure 12.3	See Table 12.1

POINTS	MERIDIAN NUMBER	CONDITIONS HELPED
8 Qu Qi	LI 11. See Figure 12.2	See Table 12.2

Please refer to the accompanying Figures (illustrations) for the locations of the points. And please note that these illustrations are for information only and may not show all the exact locations of the acupuncture points.

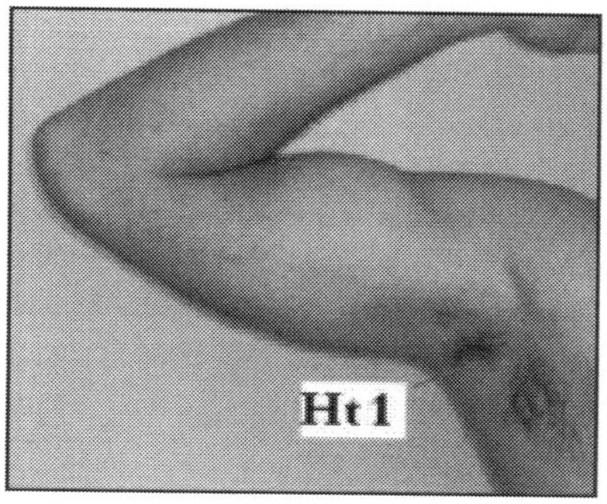

FIGURE 26.7

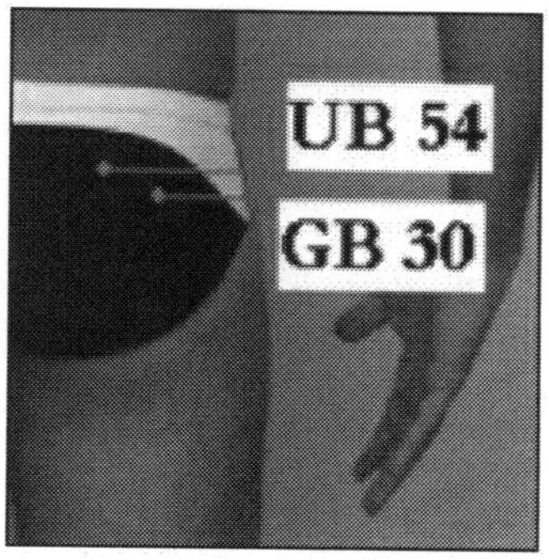

FIGURE 26.8

Acupuncture Treatments for Facial Paralysis of the Central Type

In this type, the facial paralysis is secondary to a brain stroke. The person's eye is unable to close, the tongue extends to the stroke side, and there is difficulty opening or closing the mouth, which may

TABLE 26.3

POINTS	MERIDIAN NUMBER	CONDITIONS HELPED
1 Feng Chi	GB 20. See Figure 22.4	See Table 22.1
2 Tai Yang	EX–HN 5. See Figure 15.2	Headaches, eye diseases, off –center deviation of the eyes and mouth
3 Jia Guan	St 7. See Figure 26.9	Deafness, tinnitus, toothache, facial paralysis, face pain, jaw impairment
4 Di Chang	St 4. See Figure 26.9	Off–center deviation of the mouth, salivation, twitching eyelids
5 Jia Che	St 6. See Figure 26.9	Facial paralysis, toothache, swelling of the cheek and face, mumps, spasms of jaw muscles
6 He Cu	LI 4. See Figure 12.3	See Table 12.1

Please refer to the accompanying Figures (illustrations) for the locations of the points. And please note that these illustrations are for information only and may not show all the exact locations of the acupuncture points.

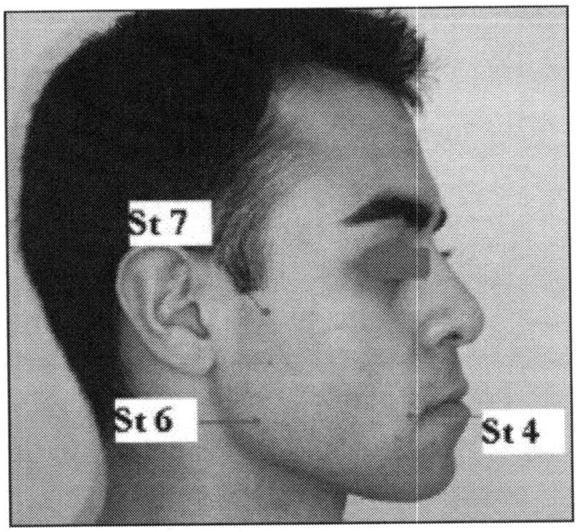

FIGURE 26.9

be drooping. The following points are used with this type of facial paralysis.

- Body Points: GB 20 Feng Chi, Ex-HN 5 Tai Yang, St 7 Xia Guan, St 4 Di Chang penetrate to St 6 Jia Che, and LI 4 He Gu for the healthy side.
- Scalp points: Lan 1, S3.

Acupuncture Treatments for Language Deficit

When there is a language deficit, the person can understand instructions, but cannot answer questions; or the person can speak, but cannot understand instructions; or the person can neither understand instructions nor speak correctly. The following points are used with language deficits.

- Body points: D 23 Shang Xin penetrate to D 20 Bai Hui, GB 20 Feng Chi, Ex-HN 3 Ying Tang, Ex-HN 12 Jin Jin, Ex-HN 13 Yu Ye, Ht 5 Tong Li, UB 10 Tian Zhu, and Ren 23 Lian Quan.
- Scalp points: Lan 1, Lan 2, and Lan 3.

TABLE 26.4

POINTS	MERIDIAN NUMBER	CONDITIONS HELPED
1 Shang Xin	Du 23. See Figure 29.3	See Table 29.2
2 Bai Hui	Du 20. See Figure 16.4	See Table 16.2
3 Feng Chi	GB 20. See Figure 22.4	See Table 22.1

POINTS	MERIDIAN NUMBER	CONDITIONS HELPED
4 Ying Tang	Ex–HN 3 22.1	See Table 22.2
5 Jin Jin/Yu Ye	Ex–HN 12/13. See Figure 26.10	Swelling of the tongue, vomiting, aphasia with stiffness of tongue
6 Tong Li	Ht 5. See Figure 26.13	Palpitations, dizziness, blurred vision, sore throat, sudden loss of voice, aphasia with stiffness of the tongue, pain in wrist and elbow
7 Tian Zhu	UB 10. See Figure 26.12	Headaches, nasal obstruction, sore throat, neck rigidity, pain in the shoulder and back
8 Lian Quan	Ren 23. See Figure 26.11	Swelling and pain of subglossal region (below the tongue), salivation with speech difficulty, non–speech with stiffness of tongue, hoarse voice, difficulty swallowing

Please refer to the accompanying Figures (illustrations) for the locations of the points. And please note that these illustrations are for information only and may not show all the exact locations of the acupuncture points.

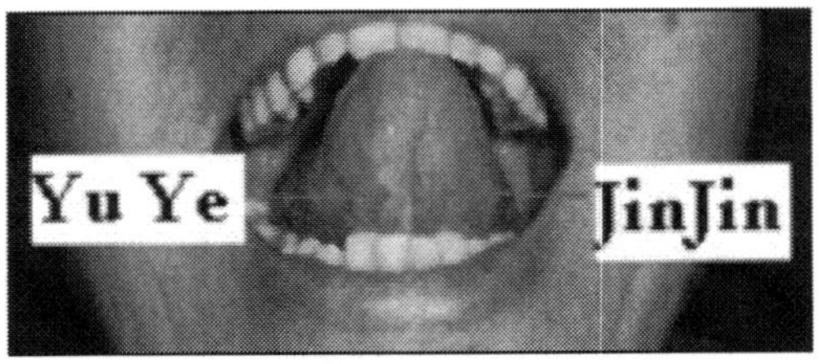

FIGURE 26.10

Acupuncture Treatments for Upper Arm Paralysis

Symptoms of this type of stroke are weakness and an inability to extend the elbow, wrist, and fingers. The following points are used with upper arm paralysis.

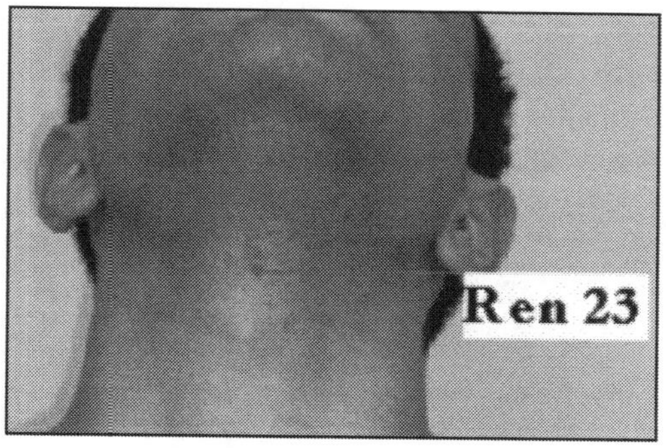

FIGURE 26.11

- Body points: GB 20 Feng Chi, Ht 1 Ji Quan, Lu 5 Qi Zhe, LI 4 He Gu, LI 15 Jian Yu, LI 11 Qu Qi, and SJ 5 Wai Guan.
- Scalp points: M 2 and M 3.

TABLE 26.5

POINTS	MERIDIAN NUMBER	CONDITIONS HELPED
1 Feng Chi	GB 20. See Figure 22.4	See Table 22.1
2 Ji Quan	Ht 1. See Figure 26.7	See Table 26.2
3 Qi Zhe	Lu 5. See Figure 13.2	See Table 13.2
4 He Gu	LI 4. See Figure 12.3	See Table 12.1

POINTS	MERIDIAN NUMBER	CONDITIONS HELPED
5 Jian Yu	1-1 15. See Figure 26.6	Shoulder and arm pain, motor impairment of the upper extremities, German measles, skin disease
6 Qu Qi	LI 11. See Figure 12.2	See Table 12.2
7 Wai Guan	SJ S. See Figure 1	2.3 See Table 12.2

Please refer to the accompanying Figures (illustrations) for the locations of the points. And please note that these illustrations are for information only and may not show all the exact locations of the acupuncture points.

Acupuncture Treatments for Shoulder Pain and Frozen Shoulder

Symptoms include difficulty raising shoulder, limited range of motion, difficulty combing hair, putting on a bra, and inserting the arm into a sleeve. The following points are used for shoulder pain and frozen shoulder.

- Body points: LI 15 Jian Yu, Du 26 Ren Zhong, SI 9 Jian Zhen, SI 15 Jian Zhong Shu, SI 14 Jian Wai Shu, and St 38 Tiao Kou.
- Scalp points: M 2 and M 3.

TABLE 26.6

POINTS	MERIDIAN NUMBER	CONDITIONS HELPED
1 Jian Yu	LI 15. See Figure 26.6	See Table 26.5
2 Ren Zhong	Du 26. See Figure 29.3	See Table 29.2
3 Jian Zhen	SI 9. See Figure 26.16	Pain in the shoulder area, impairment of hands and arms
4 Jian Zhong Shu	SI 15. See Figure 26.16	Cough, asthma, pain in the shoulder and back

POINTS	MERIDIAN NUMBER	CONDITIONS HELPED
5 Jian Wai Shu	SI 14. See Figure 26.16	Aching shoulder and back, neck pain and rigidity
6 Tiao Kou	St 38. See Figure 26.14	Numbness, soreness and pain of the knee and leg, weakness and impairment of the foot, pain and impairment of the shoulder, abdominal pain

Please refer to the accompanying Figures (illustrations) for the locations of the points. And please note that these illustrations are for information only and may not show all the exact locations of the acupuncture points.

Acupuncture Treatments for Lower Extremity Paralysis

Symptoms include weakness, difficulty lifting leg, and walking. The following points are used for lower extremity paralysis.

- Body points: UB 40 Wei Zhong, Sp 6 San Ying Jiao, GB 30 Huan Tiao, GB 34 Yang Ling Quan, and UB 60 Kun Lun.
- Scalp points: M 1 and M 2.

TABLE 26.7

POINTS	MERIDIAN NUMBER	CONDITIONS HELPED
1 Wei Zhong	UB 40. See Figure 26.8	Low back pain, motor impairment of the hip joint, hemiplegia (paralysis), pain, numbness, and motor impairment of the lower extremities, abdominal pain, vomiting
2 San Ying Jiao	Sp 6. See Figure 16.6	See Table 16.1
3 Huan Tiao	GB 30. See Figure 26.8	Pain of the lumbar region and thigh, muscular atrophy of the lower limbs

POINTS	MERIDIAN NUMBER	CONDITIONS HELPED
4 Yang Ling Quan	GB 34. See Figure 15.3	See Table 15.3
5 Kun Lun	UB 60. See Figure 26.14	Headaches, blurred vision, neck rigidity, nosebleed, shoulder, back, and arm pain, swelling and pain of the heel, difficult labor, epilepsy

Please refer to the accompanying Figures (illustrations) for the locations of the points. And please note that these illustrations are for information only and may not show all the exact locations of the acupuncture points.

Acupuncture Treatments for Poor Balance and Unsteady Gait

The following points are used for poor balance and an unsteady gait.

- Body points: GB 19 Nao Kong penetrating to GB 20 Feng Chi, UB 9 Yu Zhen penetrating to UB 10 Tian Zhu, Du 17 Nao Hu penetrating to Du 16 Feng Fu, and GB 20 Feng Chi.
- Scalp points: Balance area.

TABLE 26.8

POINTS	MERIDIAN NUMBER	CONDITIONS HELPED
1 Nao Kong	GB 19. See Figure 26.12	Headaches, stiffness of the neck, vertigo, painful eyes, tinnitus, epilepsy
2 Feng Chi	GB 20. See Figure 22.4	See Table 22.1
3 Yu Zhen	UB 9. See Figure 26.12	Headaches and neck pain, dizziness, pain in the eye, nasal obstruction

POINTS	MERIDIAN NUMBER	CONDITIONS HELPED
4 Tian Zhu	UB 10. See Figure 26.12	Headaches, nasal obstruction, sore throat, neck rigidity, pain in the shoulder and back
5 Nao Hu	Du 17. See Figure 26.12	Epilepsy, dizziness, pain and stiffness of the neck
6 Feng Fu	Du 16. See Figure 26.12	Headaches, neck rigidity, blurred vision, nosebleed, sore throat, mental disorders

Please refer to the accompanying Figures (illustrations) for the locations of the points. And please note that these illustrations are for information only and may not show all the exact locations of the acupuncture points.

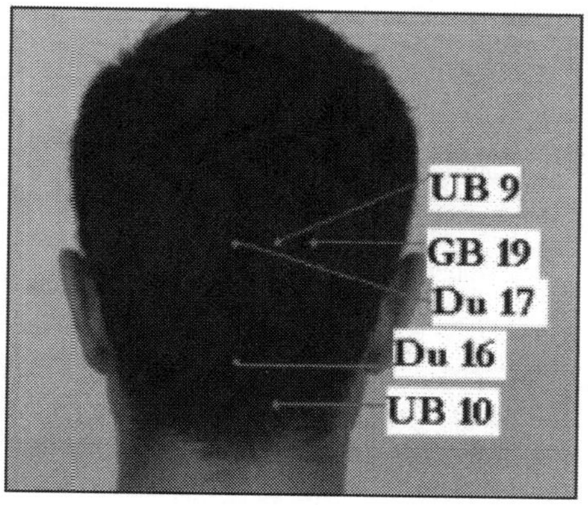

FIGURE 26.12

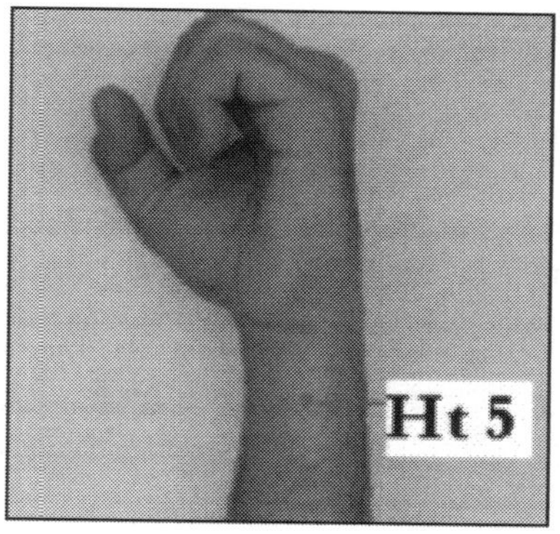

FIGURE 26.13

Acupuncture Treatments for Blindness

The following points are used for blindness.

- Body points: GB 20 Feng Chi and UB 10 Tian Zhu.
- Scalp points: Vision area.

TABLE 26.9

POINTS	MERIDIAN NUMBER	CONDITIONS HELPED
1 Feng Chi	GB 20. See Figure 22.4	See Table 22.1
2 Tian Zhu	UB 10. See Figure 26.12	Headaches, nasal obstruction, sore throat, neck rigidity, pain in the shoulder and back

Please refer to the accompanying Figures (illustrations) for the locations of the points. And please note that these illustrations are for information only and may not show all the exact locations of the acupuncture points.

Acupuncture Treatments for Difficulty Swallowing

The following points are used for difficulty in swallowing.

- Body points: PC 6 Nei Guan, Du 26 Ren Zhong, GB 20 Feng Chi, and Ren 23 Lian Quan.
- Scalp points: M 2 and M 3.

Acupuncture Treatments for Constipation

The following points are used for constipation.

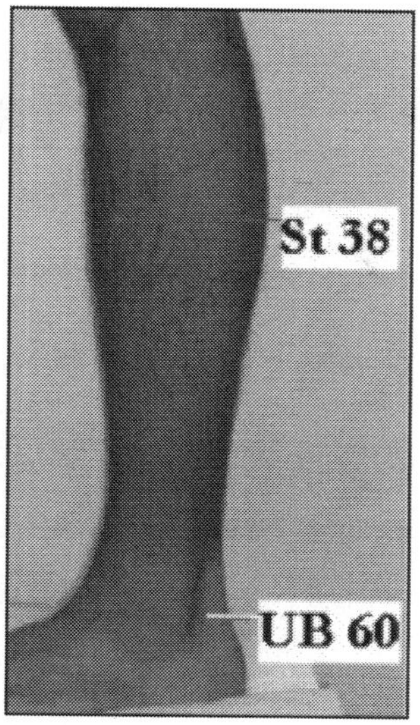

FIGURE 26.14

TABLE 26.10

POINTS	MERIDIAN NUMBER	CONDITIONS HELPED
1 Nei Guang	PC 6. See Figure 16.7	See Table 16.1
2 Ren Zhong	Du 26. See Figure 29.3	See Table 29.2
3 Feng Chi	GB 20. See Figure 22.4	See Table 22.1
4 Lian Quan	Ren 23. See Figure 26.11	Swelling and pain of subglossal region (below the tongue), salivation with speech difficulty, non–speech with stiffness of tongue, hoarse voice, difficulty swallowing

Please refer to the accompanying Figures (illustrations) for the locations of the points. And please note that these illustrations are for information only and may not show all the exact locations of the acupuncture points.

- Body points: St 40 Feng Long, St 28 Shui Dao, and St 29 Gui Lai.
- Scalp points: M 2 and M 3.

TABLE 26.11

POINTS	MERIDIAN NUMBER	CONDITIONS HELPED
1 Feng Long	St 40. See Figure 13.4	Headaches, dizziness, cough, asthma, excessive sputum, chest pain, constipation, epilepsy, muscular atrophy, motor impairment, pain, swelling, or paralysis of lower extremities
2 Shui Dao	St 28. See Figure 26.15	Retention of urine, swelling, hernia, painful menstruation
3 Gui Lai	St 29. See Fiqure 26.15	Abdominal pain, hernia, painful, irregular menstruation , absence of menstruation, white vaginal discharge, collapsed uterus

Please refer to the accompanying Figures (illustrations) for the locations of the points. And please note that these illustrations are for information only and may not show all the exact locations of the acupuncture points.

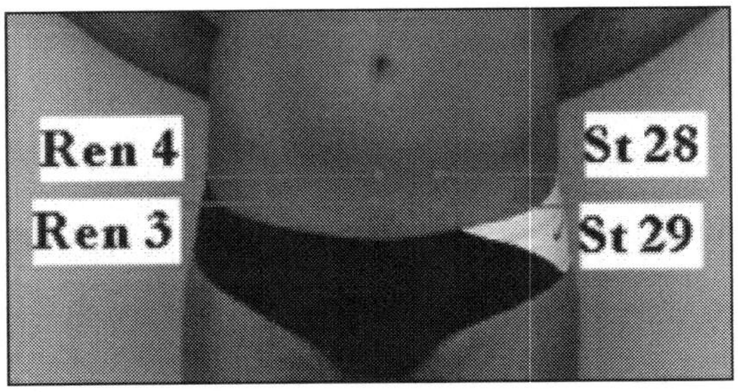

FIGURE 26.15

Acupuncture Treatments for Stoppage of Urine Flow

The following points are used for stoppage of urine flow.

- Body points: UB 54 Zhi Bian penetrate to St 28 Shui Dao, and Ren 3 Zhong Ji.
- Scalp points: M 2 and M 3.

TABLE 26.12

POINTS	MERIDIAN NUMBER	CONDITIONS HELPED
1 Zhi Bian	UB 54. See Figure 26.8	Low back pain, muscular atrophy, motor impairment of the lower extremities, painful urination, swelling around external genitalia, hemorrhoids, constipation
2 Shui Dao	St 28. See Figure 26.15	Hernia, swelling, painful menstruation, urine retention
3 Zhong Ji	Ren 3. See Figure 26.15	Bedwetting, nocturnal emissions, impotence, hernia, uterine bleeding, irregular menstruation, frequency of urination, retention of urine, pain collapse of uterus, in the lower abdomen, vaginitis

Please refer to the accompanying Figures (illustrations) for the locations of the points. And please note that these illustrations are for information only and may not show all the exact locations of the acupuncture points.

Acupuncture Treatments for Urinary Incontinence

The following points are used for urinary incontinence.

- Body points: Ren 4 Guan Yuan, Ren 6 Qi Hai, and Ki 3 Tai Xi.
- Scalp points: M 2 and M 3

TABLE 26.13

POINTS	MERIDIAN NUMBER	CONDITIONS HELPED
1 Guan Yuan	Ren 4. See Figure 26.15	Bedwetting, frequency of urination, retention of urine, hernia, irregular menstruation, uterine bleeding, postpartum hemorrhage, lower abdominal pain, indigestion, diarrhea, collapse of rectum
2 Qi Hai	Ren 6. See Figure 26.15	Abdominal pain, bedwetting, impotence, hernia, swelling, diarrhea, dysentery, uterine bleeding, irregular menstruation, white vaginal discharge, postpartum hemorrhage, constipation, asthma
3 Tai Xi	Ki 3. See Figure 14.5	See Table 14.4

WILLIAM'S TREATMENT

William underwent my treatment for two months, after which his muscle strength gradually improved to the point that he could move his shoulders, elbows, hips, and knees. By constantly flexing these joints, he had no problem with flexion and extension movements in them, but he still needed treatment for muscle strength and range of motion in the wrists and ankles. For these, he came in two to three times a week for eight weeks, then only once a week for ten weeks, at which time he was also given physical therapy to help muscle strength and range of motion for the upper and lower extremities. All these treatments helped William immensely.

Stroke treatment by acupuncture focuses on the brain and blood supply. Since the main cause of a stroke is a decreased supply of blood to the brain in either ischemic or hemorrhagic strokes, replenishing the brain's blood supply greatly improves the functions of the paralyzed parts of the body. It is necessary to treat not only the upper and lower extremities, but also the brain, or the person will be at a functional disadvantage. Thus the combination of treatments works best for anyone who has had a stroke.

A combination of acupuncture, therapy, and therapeutic massage, done together, is the best hope for totally recovering from a stroke.

TIPS FOR PEOPLE WHO HAVE HAD A STROKE

- You should ask your acupuncturist to perform the acupuncture treatments for both the body and the scalp.
- The earlier you seek out acupuncture treatment, the better your chances for recovery.
- Always try to fight the effects of the stroke by not using your unaffected extremity, but instead forcing yourself to use the paralyzed part.
- The combination of acupuncture, physical therapy, therapeutic massage, and self-motivated exercise is the best approach for recovery.

27

Bell's Palsy

JOAN'S NUMBNESS

Joan S, a forty-five-year-old woman, awoke one morning to find that when she brushed her teeth she felt numbness on the left side of her face. Her left eye was dry and she had difficulty closing it, plus her mouth tasted odd and she could not hold water in it. When she realized she was drooling, and began to feel that the left side of her face was paralyzed, she immediately called her husband who arranged for an ambulance to take her to the hospital, where she was given a CT scan and an MRI of the brain. The results showed she had not suffered a stroke, but during the physical examination she felt dizzy and realized she was again drooling out the left side of her mouth. She had a dry mouth, her left facial muscles were twitching, she was hypersensitive to sound, and she had developed slurred speech. The doctors diagnosed her condition as Bell's Palsy and gave her a corticosteroid patch for ten days, decreasing the dosage daily. When there was no improvement after the ten-day treatment, she consulted her primary care physician who prescribed acyclovir, which was supposed to prevent further damaging of the facial nerve.

After a week of acyclovir, she still felt no improvement, so she returned to this same doctor and he said her symptoms should disappear spontaneously within three to six months. After three months of no improvement, she became extremely frustrated with her condition. She still felt numbness on the left side of her face and had difficulty closing her eyes and mouth, which were both drooping; she was drooling and could not smile using the left side of her mouth. Once again back with the same doctor, he advised her that things should right themselves if she gave it more time. At this point, Joan started to feel scared, so she asked around and was referred to me by her friends.

Joan's condition, Bell's Palsy, is a form of temporary facial paralysis resulting from damage or trauma to cranial nerve VII, one of the two facial nerves. This paralysis causes muscle distortion and interferes with such facial functions as closing the eyes, eating, and using one side of the mouth. The onset of Bell's Palsy is usually sudden—many people wake up one morning to discover that one side of their face is paralyzed. Sometimes the symptoms are confused with a stroke, but Bell's Palsy is definitely not a stroke, it is only due to injury to the cranial nerve VII.

FUNCTIONS OF CRANIAL NERVE VII

- Cranial nerve VII has many nerve fibers, which are distributed to the scalp, the face, and the facial muscles. It supplies some of the salivary glands, which provide lubricants to the eyes and mouth and is responsible for sensations to the hearing organs—the ear canal and behind the ear.
- Its nerve fibers affect the forehead and the upper eyelids, including eyebrow elevation, forehead wrinkling, frowning, and tight closing of the eyes.
- Its nerve fibers in the lower face include showing the teeth, whistling, puffing the cheeks, and having a natural smile; it is also responsible for impulses to two-thirds of the tongue, including the ability to taste.

DISCOVERY, SYMPTOMS, AND CAUSES OF BELL'S PALSY

The disease is named for Sir Charles Bell, a Scottish surgeon who discovered the nerve and its effects on the facial muscles about 200 years ago. It affects about 40,000 people in the United States each year, and is most commonly seen in young adults.

Many people think it is an inflammation and swelling of the facial nerve that leads to an the onset of Bell's Palsy. This condition can be triggered by a virus infection, such as chicken pox, herpes simplex, herpes zoster, HIV, mononucleosis, or mumps, or by a bacterial infection, such as Lyme disease or tuberculosis. Others believe that brain-stem tumors, skull fractures, or neurological conditions, such as diabetic neuropathy or Guillain-Barre syndrome, can lead to Bell's Palsy.

The most common symptoms are the sudden onset of paralysis or weakness of one side of the face, with difficulty closing the eyes, facial droop and difficulty with facial expressions, pain behind or in front of the ear with an amplification of sounds on the affected side, headache, loss of taste, and changes in the amount of tears and saliva.

TREATMENTS IN WESTERN MEDICINE

The treatment of Bell's Palsy is controversial in Western medicine; many people are given no treatment and are expected to recover spontaneously. Some Western doctors prescribe the following treatments.

- **Medications.** The one most usually prescribed is a corticosteroid, sometimes mixed with antiviruses, such as acyclovir, which are expected to help in recovery.
- **Physical therapy.** It is believed that physical therapy can relax the strain in the facial muscle and prevent the symptoms from recurring.

- **Surgery.** Surgery is very controversial. If the facial paralysis has not recovered after 6 months, a person can manifest many symptoms, including drooping eyes and difficulty closing them, and distortion and spasms of the facial muscles. Although such surgical procedures as facial nerve repair, facial nerve graft, facial nerve substitution, and muscle transposition are not able to completely restore normal function, they can significantly improve the face's appearance and ability to function.

In Joan's case, her primary care doctor thought medication alone would be sufficient treatment, so she waited three of the six months he suggested without becoming better. It was at this point that she decided to consult me.

TREATMENTS IN TRADITIONAL CHINESE MEDICINE

Traditional Chinese medicine believes that facial paralysis is due to wind invasion. The wind attacks the facial nerve and causes nerve and muscle paralysis. Because the nerve supplies the impulses to the facial muscle, the taste buds, and the eye, paralysis causes muscle dysfunction and makes treatment of acupuncture at the appropriate points most important. And the sooner treatment starts, the better. It is not good to wait six months, or even three, as Joan did, to see if there is a spontaneous recovery; it is best to start treatment immediately because the viability of the facial nerve decreases every day. Even after six months, there is still a good chance of recovering from the paralysis, but instead of waiting that long, it is better to treat the affected person as soon as possible.

People with Bell's Palsy are almost always nervous about their condition, and feel extremely stressed, believing their symptoms could be the signs of a stroke. For this reason, the acupuncture treatment should not only treat the paralysis, but also utilize points intended to relieve stress.

The following points used for this condition are locally selected—most of them are on the face.

Yang Bai penetrating Yu Yao, and Si Bai, Tai Yang penetrating Xia Guan, Di Chang penetrating Jia Che, Ying Xiang, Zhuan Zhu, Cheng Jian, Feng Chi, Yi Feng, and He Gu.

TABLE 27.1

POINTS	MERIDIAN NUMBER	CONDITIONS HELPED
1 Yang Bai	GB 14. See Figure 27.1	Frontal headaches, eye pain, vertigo, twitching or drooping eyelids, tearing up
2 Yu Yao	Ex–HN 4. See Figure 27.1	Pain above the eye, twitching or drooping eyelids, cloudiness of the cornea, redness, swelling, and pain in the eye

POINTS	MERIDIAN NUMBER	CONDITIONS HELPED
3 Si Bai	St 2. See Figure 27.1	Redness, pain, and itching of the eyes, facial paralysis, twitching eyelids, pain in the face
4 Tai Yang	Ex–HN 5. See Figure 15.2	See Table 15.2
5 Xia Guan	St 7. See Figure 26.9	See Table 26.3
6 Di Chang	St 4. See Figure 26.9	See Table 26.3
7 Jia Che	St 6. See Figure 26.9	See Table 26.3
8 Ying Xiang	LI 20. See Figure 27.1	Nasal obstruction, smell impairment, itching and swelling of the face
9 Zan Zhu	UB 2. See Figure 27.1	Headaches, blurred and failing vision, pain in the ridge above the eye, tearing, redness, swelling and pain of the eye, twitching of eyelids, glaucoma
10 Chen Jiang	Ren 24. See Figure 27.1	Facial puffiness, swelling of the gums, toothache, salivation, mental disorders
11 Feng Chi	GB 20. See Figure 22.4	See Table 22.1
12 I Y Feng	SI 1 7. See Figure 25.1	See Table 25.1
13 He Cu	LI 4. See Figure 12.2	See Table 12.1

Please refer to the accompanying Figures (illustrations) for the locations of the points. And please note that these illustrations are for information only and may not show all the exact locations of the acupuncture points.

JOAN'S TREATMENT

Joan was treated with the above acupuncture points, which helped supply the blood flow to the nerve and decreased the muscle spasms and inflammation. She also received massages, and after one month of these treatments she completely recovered from Bell's Palsy.

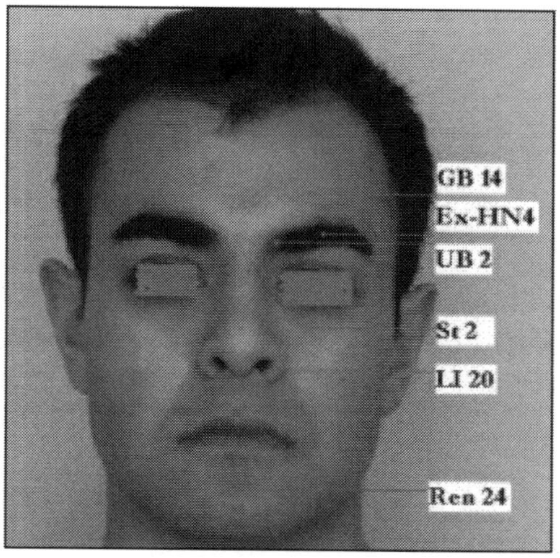

FIGURE 27.1

TIPS FOR PEOPLE WITH BELL'S PALSY

- I cannot stress enough the importance of treatment as soon as possible; waiting is not an option.
- Daily massages, 20 minutes per session and 3 sessions per day, combined with the above acupuncture points, will greatly help recovery. Acupressure the points with your thumb or knuckle, pressing with comfortable pressure on the points; count to 20, then change to another point. You should work symmetric points at the same time.

28

Restless Leg Syndrome

LUAN'S NUMBNESS AND TINGLING

Luan W is a forty-three-year-old woman who experienced restless leg syndrome for five months before she came to me. She had severe stress from both her job and her family life and began to feel numbness and tingling in both her legs along with a kind of electrical shock. She had the feeling of ants running up and down both legs, and this became particularly uncomfortable when she was sitting down or going to the bathroom. Because of the stress, LuAn had difficulty falling asleep and felt the urge to move her legs frequently during the night. As the symptoms got worse, she was unable to sleep at all as she constantly had to move her legs. She consulted her primary care physician and he referred her to a neurologist who prescribed Requip for a month and a half. When this did not produce any improvement, he tried Neupro, a transdermal patch, which made her a little better, but whenever she felt stress she slept poorly and had some depression, so she came to me for evaluation and treatment.

My examination did not indicate anything wrong; LuAn, a very pleasant woman, felt tired much of the time and was experiencing stress and depression, with poor sleep and a bad appetite. Her primary care physician sent over her blood tests, which were normal, and we both determined that her problem was restless leg syndrome.

TYPES OF RESTLESS LEG SYNDROME

There are two types of restless leg syndrome.

- **Primary restless leg syndrome** is usually considered idiopathic (from unknown causes) and hereditary. Many people think it is related to stress, though this is not strictly accurate. Stress will not cause this condition, though it can aggravate it, as will pregnancy or hormonal changes.
- **Secondary restless leg syndrome.** There are many reasons for this, but the most common are below.

  * Iron deficiency, caused by such conditions as GI bleeding or a heavy menstrual period, can cause or worsen the condition.

  * Peripheral neuropathy, a condition related to diabetes or alcoholism, can cause numbness, tingling, and a needle-like sensation in the legs, which may trigger or worsen restless leg syndrome.

  * It can also be caused by Parkinson's disease or certain autoimmune disorders, such as celiac disease, diabetes, folate deficiency, hypoglycemia, hypothyroidism, rheumatoid arthritis, Sjogren's syndrome, sleep apnea, thyroid disease, or varicose veins.

TREATMENTS IN WESTERN MEDICINE

For secondary restless leg syndrome, use iron compensate as a treatment for the causes listed above.

- **Medication.** In 2005, the FDA approved the use of ropinrole, which is a dopamine agonist used to treat moderate to severe restless leg syndrome. Its mechanism of action is to stimulate dopamine receptors, and it was initially approved for the treatment of Parkinson's disease. In 2006, the FDA approved pramipexole and, in 2007, rotigotine for RLS.
- **Other medications** such as opioids, benzodiazepine, anticonvulsants, or carbamazepine, are also used; they have different results, with some people feeling better, but others not improving at all.

TREATMENTS IN TRADITIONAL CHINESE MEDICINE

Many recent studies show that impaired functioning of the musculoskeletal system might be the cause of restless leg syndrome, therefore acupuncture treatment focuses on the dysfunction. Two types of needles are used.

- The needles on the top of the scalp for the points that act on the brain system and the central nervous system, such as Si Shen Chong, GB 8 Shuai Gu, and Du20 Bai Hui. This needle placement will increase endorphine and dopamine secretions, which decrease stress and depression.

- Needles on the legs for the second group of points are Sp 9 Ying Ling Quin, GB 34 Yang Ling Quan, St 36 Zu San Li, and Sp 6 San Yin Jiao. These points on the leg adjust the meridians' secretions and improve the nutritional supply to the legs. This is very effective in decreasing the symptoms of restless leg syndrome.

TABLE 28.1

POINTS	MERIDIAN NUMBER	CONDITIONS HELPED
1 Si Sheng Chong	Ex–HN 1. See Figure 28.1	Headaches, vertigo, insomnia, poor memory, epilepsy
2 Shui Gu	GB 8. See Figure 22.1	See Table 22.6
3 Bai Hui	Du 20. See Figure 16.4	See Table 16.2
4 Ying Ling Quan	Sp 9. See Figure 28.2	Abdominal pain, diarrhea, dysentery, swelling, jaundice, incontinence, pain in the external genitalia, pain in the knee
5 Yang Ling Quan	GB 34. See Figure 15.3	See Table 15.3
6 Zu San Li	St 36. See Figure 13.4	See Table 13.3
7 San Yin Jiao	Sp 6. See Figure 16.6	See Table 16.1

Please refer to the accompanying Figures (illustrations) for the locations of the points. And please note that these illustrations are for information only and may not show all the exact locations of the acupuncture points.

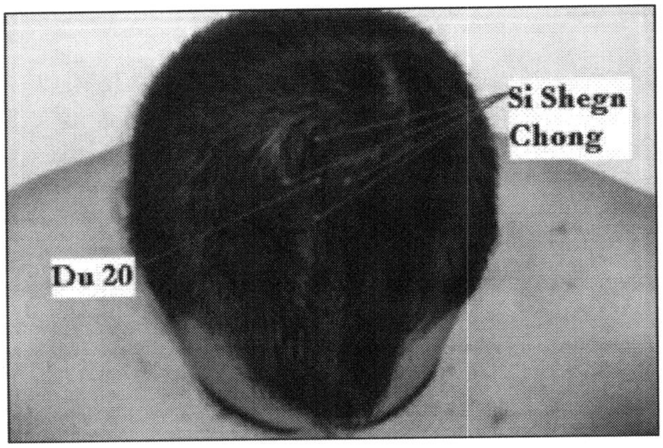

FIGURE 28.1

LUAN'S TREATMENT

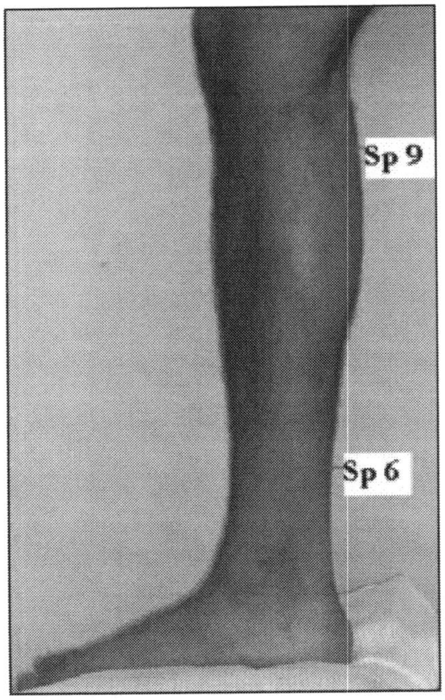

FIGURE 28.2

LuAn underwent acupuncture treatments for fifteen visits and, at the same time reduced her stress by taking a new job. She also managed to resolve her family issue, so with the acupuncture treatments she was able to get better sleep and felt much more relaxed and less depressed. This, in turn, reduced the leg numbness and tingling sensation in her legs, and her restless leg syndrome is much improved.

I have come across many physicians who do not think restless leg syndrome is related to stress. However, the combination of treating for stress at the same time as treating for restless leg syndrome seems more effective than treating the syndrome alone.

In treating LuAn, it was necessary to put her in an isolated room with a relaxed environment of music and semi-darkness for thirty minutes, and utilize a heating pad along with the acupuncture needles.

As was the case with LuAn, these treatments should be given three times a week for four to six weeks. For the first few visits, the person being treated may not feel any improvement, but after five or six visits she will usually feel great improvement and will not need to move her legs as much as before.

TIP FOR PEOPLE WITH RESTLESS LEG SYNDROME

- Magnesium deficiency can make muscles go into spasms easily. If the amounts of body magnesium are low, you can have restless legs (among other problems). Magnesium supplementation can help stop the twitching, and a particularly effective form is Natural Vitality's CALM. A teaspoon or more of this powder taken daily works best when dissolved and drunk in filtered hot water.

MAGNESIUM AND CALCIUM

Magnesium is a fundamental nutrient that needs to be in balance with calcium in order to fully experience good health. Calcium and magnesium are like opposite sides of a coin. Calcium excites nerves, while magnesium calms them down. Calcium makes muscles contract; magnesium is necessary for muscles to relax. Calcium is needed for blood clotting, but magnesium keeps the blood flowing freely.

Progressive Health Neutraceuticals Website: www.progressivehealth.com/RLS-magnesium.asp

29

Bipolar Disorder

MARY'S MOOD SWINGS

Mary S, a seventy-two-year-old woman who has a long history of depression and manic disorder, was brought to my office by her husband. He reported that, for over a week, she had been lying on her bed staring at the ceiling, without speaking or having any facial expression. He told me she was often in conflict with a neighbor over a property-line dispute and after any confrontation, she would take to her bed and stare at the ceiling. Mary refused to eat, speak, or go to the bathroom, though her husband forced her to eat a little of the fruit he brought her. One time, after she had been without sleep for over a week, her husband took her to a psychiatrist who found her moods to be extremely elevated at times. She was talking loudly without stopping, and was doing household tasks wildly and erratically when she was not lying in bed practically catatonic. The doctor prescribed antidepressants, giving Mary the maximum dosage possible, and when she showed no improvement, he performed twenty-seven sessions of electroshock therapy (ECT) on her over a twelve-month period.

TYPES OF BIPOLAR DISORDER

There are three types of bipolar disorder.

- Recurrent episodes of severe mania or depression.
- Milder episodes of hypomania alternating with mild depression. People in this category never experience severe mania.

ELECTROSHOCK THERAPY

ECT is one of the fastest ways to relieve symptoms of bipolar disorder when a person manifests both mania and severe depression. Prior to treatment, a muscle relaxant and general anesthesia are usually administered. An electrode is put under the scalp, then a carefully controlled electrical current is applied to the electrode and that induces a seizure attack. Because the person being treated is totally unconscious, the muscles are completely relaxed, so there is no harm to the muscles or bones. Minutes later, the person awakens, but does not remember either the treatment or the events surrounding the treatment, and is often confused.

Sometimes these ECT treatments helped Mary, sometimes not. Finally, her husband brought her in to me for evaluation and acupuncture treatment.

- Rapid-cycle bipolar disorder, which means that four or more episodes of the illness occur within a twelve-month period.

CAUSES OF BIPOLAR DISORDER

What causes bipolar disorder? There is no clear understanding of the origins and causes of the disorder, but most scientists believe there are multiple causes, which may tend to run in families. Because the same or similar DNA abnormalities were found to run in the genes of bipolar families, it is believed most likely that the combination of many different genes, acting together and in combination with other factors—such as the personal or environment factors in which a person lives—may be the cause of this illness. New technologies, such as brain imaging, MRIs, EEGs, PETs and functional MRIs, are finding more and more evidence that there are a number of different brain pathologies for people with bipolar disorder.

TREATMENTS IN WESTERN MEDICINE

According to its definition in Western medicine, bipolar disorder, formerly referred to as manic depression, is a mood disorder that causes episodes of depression and mania in mood swings that are way above and way below the normal range. At one end of the spectrum is severe depression, at the other, high elation or mania, and these mood swings are usually exhibited in very rapid succession. In a depressive episode, the person usually shows sadness, excessive loss of pleasure, abnormal sleep, restlessness, low energy, difficulty concentrating, loss of appetite, overeating, irritability, feelings of worthlessness and helplessness, and thoughts of death or suicide. However, the person can soon swing from this low point to the opposite extreme, which is characterized by extreme irritability, reckless behavior, an inappropriate sense of euphoria, talking too much, excessive energy, out-of-control spending, difficulty concentrating, and an abnormal increase of other inappropriate behavior, including sexual activity, poor judgment, and aggressive behavior.

DIAN KUANG—THE CHINESE EQUIVALENT OF BIPOLAR DISORDER

Dian kuang is a complicated disorder of the brain, and its symptoms are usually seen in youth and middle age, although they can be seen in old age as well. There are two types of dian kuang.

- Dian is associated with clumsy mental processes and an expressionless face. The person with this type is very likely depressed, remains quiet, and exhibits incoherent speech.

- Kuang can be expressed in a variety of ways: anxiety, headaches, insomnia, a fixed stare, laughing and/or anger at everyone; and sometimes the person with this type of the disorder can destroy the furniture, throw things around, and verbally abuse everyone in sight, including family members.

Many times, both types of dian and kuang are manifested at once, and the symptoms are alternated. The mixed clinical manifestations are very similar to the bipolar disorder of Western medicine.

TREATMENTS IN TRADITIONAL CHINESE MEDICINE

Dian kuang is most likely related to the heart, liver, spleen, and stomach, as well as the brain, so treatment will consist of acupuncture points associated with these organs.

Treatment for Dian

For dian, it is best to use Du, Liver, and back Shu points and meridians, such as Du 16 Feng Fu, Du 14 Da Zhui, Du 13 Tao Dao, UB 15 Xin Shu, UB 18 Gang Shu, UB 20 Pi Shu, St 40 Feng Long, Ht 7 Sheng Men, and Li 3 Tai Cong.

If the person is crying or laughing unreasonably, add PC 5 Jian Shi and Du 20 Bai Hui.

If the appetite is poor, add Ren 12 Zhong Wan and St 36 Zu San Li.

TABLE 29.1

POINTS	MERIDIAN NUMBER	CONDITIONS HELPED
1 Feng Fu	Du 16. See Figure 12.1	See Table 12.1
2 Da Zhui	Du 14. See Figure 12.1	See Table 12.2
3 Tao Dao	Du 13. See Figure 29.1	Stiff back, headaches, malaria, high fevers
4 Xin Shu	UB 15. See Figure 16.3	See Table 16.1
5 Gang Shu	UB 18. See Figure 19.1	See Table 19.3
6 Pi Shu	UB 20. See Figure 29.1	Abdominal pain and distension, jaundice, vomiting, diarrhea, dysentery, bloody stools, profuse menstruation, swelling, anorexia, back pain
7 Feng Long	St 40. See Figure	See Table 13.3
8 Sheng Men	Heart 7. See Figure 23.3	Cardiac pain, irritability, palpitations, amnesia, insomnia, epilepsy, dementia, feverish sensation in the palm
9 Tai Cong	Liver 3. See Figure 18.1	See Table 18.1
10 Jian Shi	Pericardium 5. See Figure 29.2	Cardiac pain, palpitations, stomach ache, vomiting, fevers, irritability, malaria, mental disorders, epilepsy, swelling, contractures of the elbow and arm
11 Bai Hui	Du 20. See Figure 16.4	See Table 16.2

POINTS	MERIDIAN NUMBER	CONDITIONS HELPED
12 Zhong Wan	Ren 12. See Figure 13.3	See Table 13.3
13 Zu San Li	St 36. See Figure 1 3.4	See Table 13.3

Please refer to the accompanying Figures (illustrations) for the locations of the points. And please note that these illustrations are for information only and may not show all the exact locations of the acupuncture points.

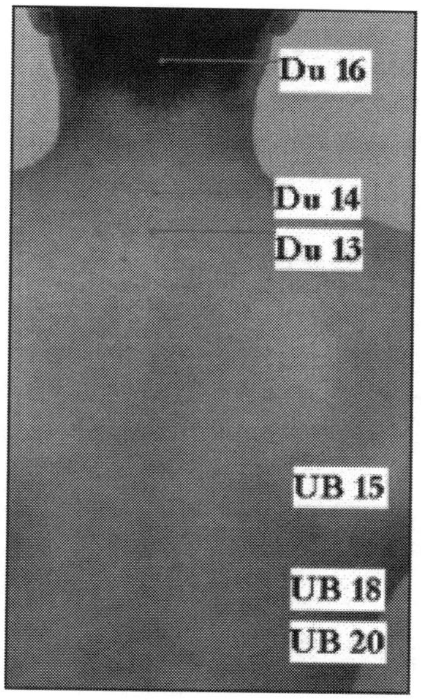

FIGURE 29.1

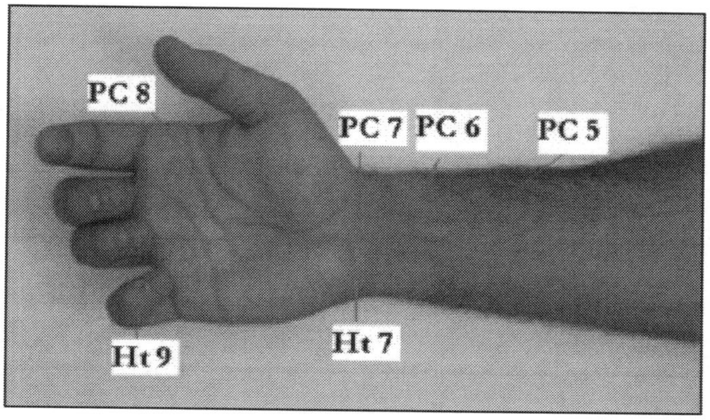

FIGURE 29.2

Treatment for Kuang

TABLE 29.2

POINTS	MERIDIAN NUMBER	CONDITIONS HELPED
1 Ren Zhong	Du 26. See Figure 29.3	Mental disorders, epilepsy, hysteria, infantile convulsion, coma, apoplexy, puffiness of the face, low back pain and stiffness
2 Shang Xin	Du 23. See Figure 29.3	Headaches, nosebleed, eye pain, runny nose, mental disorders
3 Yin Tang	Ex–HN 3. See Figure 22.2	See Table 22.1
4 Nei Guang	Pericardium 6. See Figure 16.7	See Table 16.1
5 Da Ling	Pericardium 7. See Figure 29.2	Cardiac pain, stomach ache, vomiting, mental disorders, epilepsy, stuffy chest, convulsions, insomnia, irritability, foul breath
6 Shen Mai	UB 62. See Figure 29.4	Epilepsy, mania, headaches, dizziness, insomnia, back pain, aching legs
7 Bai Hui	DU 20. See Figure 16.4	See Table 16.2
8 Tai Yang	EX–HN 5. See Figure 15.2	See Table 15.2
9 Shao Chong	Heart 9. See Figure 29.2	Palpitations, cardiac pain, pain in the chest, mania, fevers, loss of consciousness

POINTS	MERIDIAN NUMBER	CONDITIONS HELPED
10 Lao Gong	Pericardium 8. See Figure 29.2	Cardiac pain, mental disorder, epilepsy, gastritis, foul breath, fungal infection of the hand and foot, vomiting, nausea
11 Yong Quan	Kidney 1. See Figure 29.5	Headaches, blurred vision, dizziness, sore throat, dry tongue, loss of voice, loss of consciousness
12 Jian Shi	Pericardium 5. See Figure 29.1	See Table 29.1

Please refer to the accompanying Figures (illustrations) for the locations of the points. And please note that these illustrations are for information only and may not show all the exact locations of the acupuncture points.

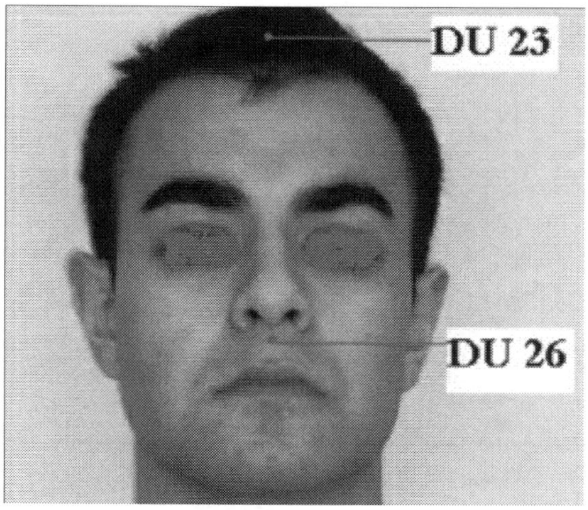

FIGURE 29.3

- For kuang it is best to use Du 26 Ren Zhong, Du 23 Shang Xin, Ex-HN3 Yin Tang, PC 6 Nei Guang, PC 7 Da Ling, and UB 52 Sheng Mai.
- If the person has a headache and insomnia, add Du 20 Bai Hui, Ex-HN 5 Tai Yang, and Ht 9 Shao Chong.

- If the person is agitated, add PC 8 Lao Gong, Ki 1 Yong Quan, and PC 5 Jian Shi.

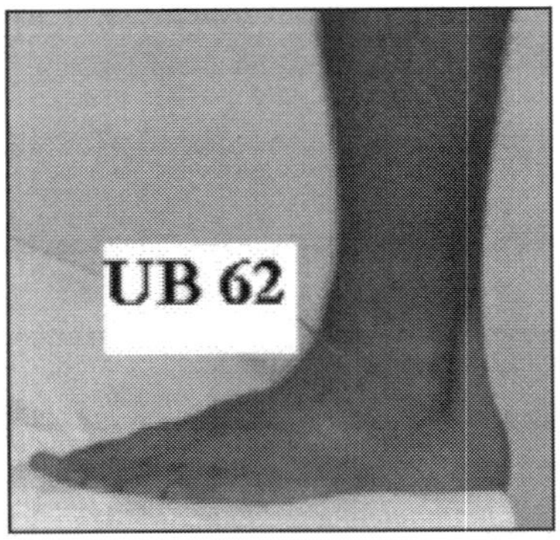

FIGURE 29.4

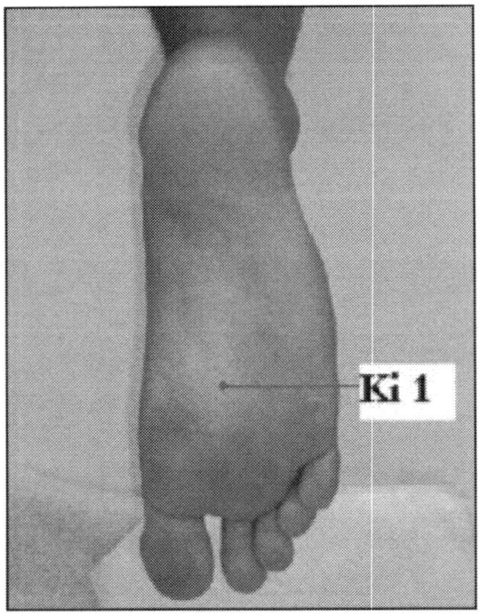

FIGURE 29.5

MARY'S TREATMENT

Mary underwent three acupuncture treatments a week for the first two months, and her symptoms gradually improved. After the two months, her treatments were cut down to twice a week and her antidepressant medication was reduced in strength. The following month, I cut her down to one acupuncture treatment a week. At this point, she was taking a very low dose of her medication and was sufficiently well to help her daughter, a hospital nurse on irregular shifts, with the care of her grandchildren. Mary enjoyed being almost normal, and was glad she could help out with the children, picking them up at school, cooking them dinner, and supervising their homework. Once a week, she delivered a cake that she had baked herself to our office. Everyone in the office, the doctor included, immensely looked forward to these cakes, and the staff regularly asked how Mary was doing and when they could expect the next cake.

TIPS FOR PEOPLE WITH BIPOLAR DISORDER

- Relax, and stick to the program.
- To calm down, massage Du 26 constantly for thirty minutes, three to four sessions per day. Acupressure the point with your thumb or knuckle, pressing with comfortable pressure on the point.

30

Unexplained infertility

AMY'S INFERTILITY

Amy S., a thirty-six-year-old woman, is an OB-GYN at a Connecticut hospital, who delivers babies every day. When she finished her residency two years ago, she and her husband wanted to have a baby and tried for a pregnancy for a year, to no avail. As a doctor, Amy is well aware of the workings of her body. She consulted the best endocrinologist and infertility specialist in the area, who checked her hormone levels, including the thyroid, pituitary gland, adrenal gland, and ovaries, only to find nothing was wrong. She was careful about nutrition, was at her ideal weight of 120 pounds, and neither drank nor smoked. She also had an ultrasound, which showed no problem in her tubes, uterus, or ovaries. Amy's husband was also examined and shown to have a normal quantity and quality of sperm with no antisperm antibodies. The delivery of his sperm was also normal; he showed no retrograde ejaculation and no blockage in the ejaculatory duct.

Amy came to me for consultation and evaluation. She is an open-minded physician, devoted to her job, and she works between fifty-five and sixty hours a week. Her husband is an emergency physician who works in the same hospital and he, too, works hard. Amy and her husband are often on call, causing much stress. They both keep irregular hours and often do not see much of each other. From her history, I could tell she was very stressed, unhelpful to her pregnancy situation.

Amy told me she had read an article which indicated that acupuncture plus IVF (in vitro fertilization) could help increase the success rate for pregnancy. She tried it once, without success.

Based on the above information, Amy has unexplained infertility. By definition, this is when a couple has not conceived after twelve months of contraceptive-free intercourse.

CAUSES OF UNEXPLAINED INFERTILITY

There are many causes of infertility.

Causes for Men

- Impaired production and function of sperm, low sperm concentration. Normal sperm concentration is greater than, or equal to, 20 million sperm per milliliter of semen. A count of 10 million or fewer sperm per milliliter of semen indicates low sperm concentration, and the chances of conception lessen. A count of 40 million sperm or higher per milliliter of semen indicates increased fertility; also, if a sperm changes its shape and mobility or is

slow, the sperm may not be able to reach or penetrate the egg.
- The malfunction of the hypothalamic-pituitary-gonadal axis; if the axis is not working properly, the male hormone level will be disturbed and the sperm will be both low in count and slow in activity.
- The testes system, including transportation and maturation.

Causes for Women

- Fallopian tube damage or blockage
- Endometriosis
- Ovulation disorders
- Early menopause
- Polycystic ovary syndrome
- Uterine fibroids

Even though there are many women who cannot conceive for any of the above reasons, there are 15 percent of couples who cannot conceive due to unexplained reasons, and Amy falls into this category.

TREATMENTS COMBINING WESTERN MEDICINE AND TCM—ACUPUNCTURE

Amy was encouraged to have IVF treatment and get acupuncture treatments beforehand. She was scheduled to have hormone treatment for a month before trying to become pregnant again, and to have acupuncture treatments with me three times a week during that month. Two groups of key acupuncture points were selected for Amy.

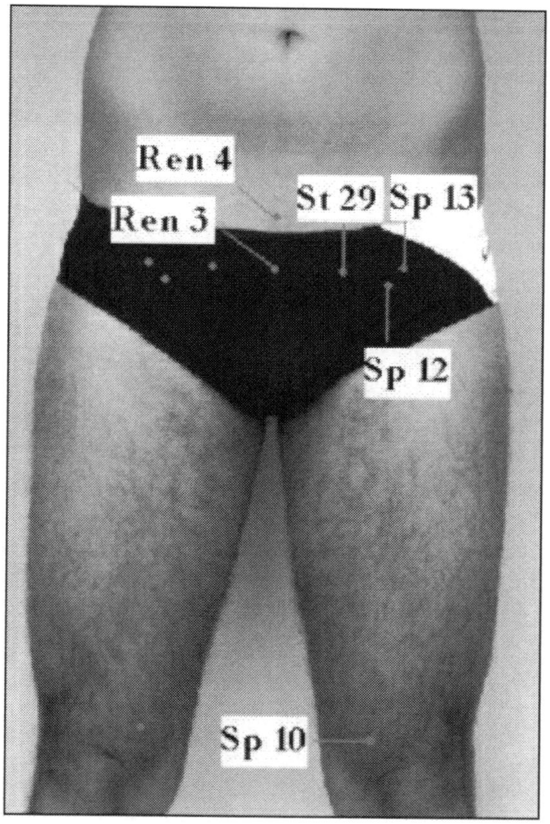

FIGURE 30.1

- Ren3 Zhong Ji, Ren4 Guang Yuan, Stomach 29 Gui Lai, Spleen 12 Chong Men, Spleen 13 Fu She. This group of acupuncture points adjusts the hormonal level of the entire body. Stimulation of the point Spleen 12 Fu she, and Spleen 13 Chong Men—both points bilateral and adjacent to the ovary and uterus—will directly adjust the ovary's hormonal secretion cycle, in turn increasing the activity of the pituitary, adrenal, and ovary axis and increasing the chance of contraception. Ren3 Zhong Ji and Ren4 Guang Yuan directly stimulate the uterus, which makes the uterus muscle very relaxed and will increase the chance of contraception and easy implantation. Stomach 29 Gui Lai is also adjacent to the ovary and uterus, and assists the first four points above in adjusting the entire female hormone system.

TABLE 30.1

POINTS	MERIDIAN NUMBER	CONDITIONS HELPED
1 Zhong Ji	Ren 3. See Figure 30.1	Problems with urination, impotence, irregular menstruation, hernia
2 Guan Yuan	Ren 4. See Figure 30.1	Nocturnal emissions, frequency of urination, retention of urine, hernia, irregular menstruation, uterine bleeding, postpartum hemorrhage, lower abdominal pain, indigestion, diarrhea, prolapse of the rectum
3 Gui Lai	St 29. See Figure 30.1	Abdominal pain, hernia, irregular menstruation, prolapse of the uterus
4 Chong Men	Sp 12. See Figure 30.1	Abdominal pain, hernia
5 Fu She	Sp 13. See Figure 30.1	Lower abdominal pain, hernia
6 He Gu	LI 4. See Figure 12.3	See Table 12.1
7 Qu Qi	U 11. See Figure 12.2	See Table 12.2

POINTS	MERIDIAN NUMBER	CONDITIONS HELPED
8 San Yin Jiao	Sp 6. See Figure 16.6	See Table 16.1
9 Xue Hai	Sp 10. See Figure 30.1	Irregular menstruation, uterine bleeding, eczema, pain in the thigh
10 Tai Chong	Sp 3. See Figure 18.2	See Table 18.1
11 Shang Liao	US 31. See Figure 30.2	Low back pain, constipation, irregular menstruation, prolapse of the uterus
12 Ci Liao	US 32. See Figure 30.2	Low back pain, hernia, irregular menstruation, nocturnal emissions, impotence, muscular atrophy, pain, numbness and motor impairment of the lower extremities
13 Zhong Liao	US 33. See Figure 30.2	Low back pain, constipation, diarrhea, irregular menstruation
14 Xia Liao	US 34. See Figure 30.2	Low back pain, lower abdominal pain, constipation

Please refer to the accompanying Figures (illustrations) for the locations of the points. And please note that these illustrations are for information only and may not show all the exact locations of the acupuncture points.

- The second group is on the back eight liao points. UB 31 Shang Liao, UB 32 Ci Liao, UB 33 Zhong Liao, UB 34 Xia Liao. Eight liao points (eight points on both sides of the sacral area, Shang Liao, Ci Liao, Zhong Liao, and Xia Liao) directly stimulate two nerves in the pelvic region. These nerves will stimulate the uterus and ovaries and thereby help to increase the chance of contraception, as well as adjust the entire hormonal system of the female reproductive system.

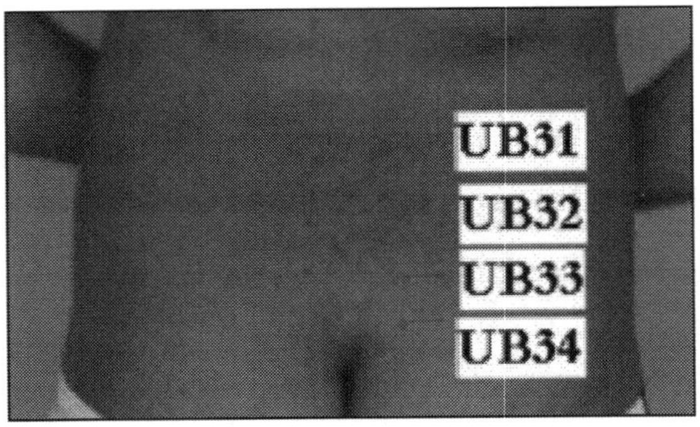

FIGURE 30.2

The two above groups of key acupuncture points were alternatively treated during each day's visit, in addition to the LI 4 He Gu, LI 11, Qu Chi, Spleen 6 San Yin Jiao, Spleen 10 Xue Hai, and Liver 3 Tai Chong, and they all helped adjust the hormonal environment in Amy's entire body and thus aid contraception.

Ater four weeks of treatment, Amy underwent the IVF procedure and was kept on the acupuncture treatment twice a week. Amy reported to me that she had eight eggs mature, an improvement from the first IVF treatment, which had produced only three mature eggs.

After a forty-eight- to seventy-two-hour culture, six of her eggs were fertilized and Amy's doctor implanted four into her uterus. The doctor told her she should have bed rest overnight and could return to work the next day. However, I told her to have two days of bed rest because Amy's job is more stressful than most people's, and she has to bend forward in her work to deliver babies.

A month after insemination, Amy told me she was pregnant. She was very excited about her condition and eight months later delivered twins, a boy and a girl. She was thrilled with the results, as was her husband.

TIPS FOR PEOPLE WITH UNEXPLAINED INFERTILITY

- In unexplained infertility, most of the cases are stress related. As an OB-GYN doctor, Amy worked very hard, as did her husband, and they had little time to be together. With both under constant stress, their bodies are always tight, in particular Amy's uterus muscles, which made it very difficult for the fertilized eggs to attach themselves to the uterus. Some women may be lucky enough to get pregnant, but they may not be able to retain their baby in the uterus because of the stress and tightness of their uteruses. They may have frequent miscarriages. My treatment is mainly for stress reduction.
- Many women with unexplained infertility have irregular hormonal environments in their bodies because of their high stress levels. These will affect their entire reproductive system, including with oocyte maturation, delivery, fertilization and implantation. My acupuncture points are selected to adjust the

hormonal environment and make the different hormones harmonious.

- Each woman should have about one month of acupuncture treatment before starting the IVF procedure in order to prepare her hormonal system and have her relax psychologically.
- It is extremely important to have forty-eight hours of bed rest after insemination before taking up normal activities because the fertilized eggs are very weakly bound to the uterus at this time. Any inappropriate movement during these first forty-eight hours might cause an early miscarriage.
- For the key acupuncture points, you may do the acupressure by yourself as indicated above. Acupressure the points with your thumb or knuckle, pressing with comfortable pressure on the points; count to 20, then change to another point. You should work symmetric points at the same time.

31

Osteoporosis

EMILY'S SEVERE OSTEOARTHRITIS

Emily M. is a fifty-nine-year-old woman. One morning, when she opened her garage to take her garbage can out to the curb, she fell and immediately felt severe pain in her right hip, which made it very difficult to get up from the ground. Her husband called 911 and Emily was taken to the ER, where an x-ray showed a fracture of the right hip that instantly required a total hip replacement because she had severe osteoporosis and her bone age, as shown by a bone scan, was equivalent to the bone age of about 80 years. After the operation, she came to my office for rehabilitation, and asked me why it was so easy to have a fracture. Her friends sometimes had falls without any problems. She wanted acupuncture treatments, and also asked for a nutritional consultation about her osteoporosis.

I asked about her past medical history and learned that when she was young, Emily was an athlete. She ran about five miles a day, five days a week for about ten years, so she was very skinny during this period. From ages sixteen to twenty-six, she rarely menstruated, but after she stopped her marathon training, she gradually recovered her menstruation. Then she got pregnant and has two children. She told me her mother also had a fall at age fifty-five and had a lumbar 4 and 5 veterbral compression fracture as well. She asked if there was any connection between her mom's fall and her own.

Emily has osteoporosis, which is often seen in women of postmenopausal age and men above age seventy-five. Osteoporosis does not usually manifest any symptoms until one day a fracture occurs. Women and men with osteoporosis most often break bones in the hip, spine, and wrist. A fracture of the bone in an older person can be a warning sign that the bone is weaker than is considered optimal. A fracture of the long bone, such as the hip and wrist, acutely impairs mobility and requires surgery. The symptoms of vertebral collapse usually include sudden back pain, often accompanied by nerve pain shooting down the legs, numbness, and a tingling sensation. This is a compression fracture and you can see the vertebral collapse in an x-ray. If there are multiple vertebral fractures, the person will have a stooped posture, loss of height, and chronic pain with reduced mobility.

RISK FACTORS FOR OSTEOPOROSIS

All post-menopausal women and men age fifty and older should be evaluated clinically for osteoporosis risk factors in order to determine the need for bone mineral density testing. Osteoporosis is preventable if the risk factors are known, so a fall causing a bone fracture can be avoided.

The Most Identifiable Risk Factors

Genetic factors. There are many genetic factors that will cause osteoporosis, such as a parental history of hip fractures, cystic fibrosis, hypophosphatasia, or idiopathic hypercalcinuria.

Lifestyle factors. These include many risk factors, such as low-calcium intake, vitamin-D insufficiency, excessive vitamin-A intake, high-caffeine intake, high-salt intake, three or more alcoholic drinks a day, immobilization, inadequate physical activity, smoking, tennis, and excessive physical activity. There are numerous examples of marathon runners who develop severe osteoporosis late in life. In women, heavy exercise can lead to decreased estrogen levels, which inhibit calcium absorption and produce osteoporosis. In addition, intensive training without proper calcium, vitamin D, and nutrition compensation will increases the risk of osteoporosis and fracture. Soft drinks, which contain phosphorus, may increase the risk of osteoporosis because the phosphoric acid will displace calcium contained in the bone.

Medications. Many medications are associated with osteoporosis and fractures.

- Glucocorticoids/steroids. If you take more than 5mg per day of prednisone or the equivalent for more than three months, it will usually cause osteoporosis.

- Anticoagulants, such as heparin.
- Anticonvulsants.
- Barbiturates.
- Chemotherapeutic drugs.
- Cyclosporin A, tacrolimus, or similar immunosuppressants.
- Lithium.

Diseases and disorders. There are many diseases associated with osteoporosis.

- Blood disorders, such as leukemia, lymphoma, multiple myeloma, or sickle cell disease.
- Endocrine disorders, such as adrenal insufficiency, Cushing's syndrome, diabetes mellitus, hyperparathyroidism, or thyrotoxicosis.
- Hypogonadal diseases, such as anorexia nervosa, Kallmann syndrome, Klinefelter syndrome, or Turner syndrome.
- Malnutrition and malabsorption, such as colitis, Crohn's disease, gastrectomy surgery, intestinal bypass surgery or bowel resection, ulcerative lactose intolerance, and vitamin-B12 or vitamin-K deficiency.
- Renal insufficiency.

WHO GETS OSTEOPOROSIS?

Osteoporosis is more common in older individuals and Caucasian women, but it can occur in men of any age, as well as women, and in all ethnic groups.

About 10 million Americans have osteoporosis, and 80 percent of these are women. One in two women has a fracture related to osteoporosis in her lifetime. Thus, women older than fifty are at the greatest risk of developing osteoporosis and experiencing related fractures.

Osteoporosis can begin at a young age if a person does not get enough calcium and vitamin D. After reaching maximum bone density and strength between the ages of twenty-five and thirty, a person loses about 0.4 percent of bone strength each year. At this rate, and with good nutrition, people should experience bone loss without developing osteoporosis.

However, after menopause, women lose bone mass at a rate that can go as high as 3 percent per year. After menopause, a women's body makes much less estrogen, a hormone substance that flows in the blood to control body functions and also helps to prevent osteoporosis. In fact, osteoporosis is common in any body that cannot make enough new bone to compensate for the body's loss of the old bone.

HOW TO DIAGNOSE OSTEOPOROSIS

The dual-energy absorptiometry (DXA) measures the hip and the spine bone density to establish or confirm the diagnosis of osteoporosis, predict future fracture risk, and monitor patients by performing serial assessments. The World Health Organization, W.H.O., has established the following definition based on BMD (bone mineral density) measurements at the spine, hip, or forearm by DXA devices.

Bone-Mineral Density (BMD)

Bone mineral density is a measured calculation of the true mass of bone. The absolute amount of bone as measured by bone mineral density (BMD) generally correlates with bone strength and its ability to bear weight. BMD cannot predict the certainty of developing a fracture; it can only predict risk. The bone densitometry test determines the bone mineral density (BMD). Your BMD is compared to two norms—healthy young adults (your T-score) and age-matched (your Z-score).

First, your BMD result is compared with the BMD results from healthy 25 to 35-year-old adults of your same sex and ethnicity. The standard deviation (SD) is the difference between your BMD and that of the healthy young adults. This result is your T-score. Positive T-scores indicate the bone is stronger than normal; negative T-scores indicate the bone is weaker than normal.

- Normal BMD is within 1 SD (Standard Deviation) of a young normal adult, T-score at 1.0 and above.
- Low bone mass osteopenia BMD is between 1.0 and 2.5 SD below that of a young normal adult, T-score between −1.0 and −2.5.
- Osteoporosis BMD is 2.5 SD or more below that of a young normal adult, T-score at or below −2.5. Those in this group who have already experienced

one or more fractures are deemed to have severe or established osteoporosis.

WHO GETS TESTED FOR BONE MINERAL DENSITY (BMD)

Based on the National Osteoporosis Foundation's *Conditions Guide,* the following people should be tested for BMD.

- Women age sixty-five and older, and men age seventy and older.
- Postmenopausal women, and men age fifty to sixty-nine when the doctor has concerns based on their risk-factor profiles.
- Anyone who has had a fracture, to determine the degree of the disease's severity.

TREATMENTS IN WESTERN MEDICINE

Prevention

Prevention is the most important treatment. The following are useful for this purpose.

Calcium. For women before menopause, 1000mg per day should be taken, and women who are postmenopausal should take 1200mg per day.

Vitamin D. 800 IU daily for women before menopause, and 1000 IU for postmenopausal women. Men up to the age of fifty should increase their vitamin D and calcium intake to 800 IU of vitamin D and 1000mg of calcium per day.

There are numerous calcium products in the market. Most of them are in tablet form, which is difficult for your body to absorb because the calcium supplement is not blended with vitamin D and magnesium, both of which are necessary to aid in the absorption and use of calcium.

Even if the calcium tablet is blended correctly, it may be difficult for the body to utilize or break down the calcium. One explanation may be that many calcium brands use calcium from eggshell or oyster shell. These may not be well absorbed by the body. Another reason calcium may not be absorbed from a tablet is because D CP, a binding agent used to hold the tablet together, does not break down in the body. In addition to binders, some calcium supplements may have additives, such as chlorine and other chemicals. Even assuming no binders are used in the calcium tablet, the body must still break a hard-pressed tablet down into a usable form. If the tablet cannot be sufficiently broken down in the stomach, then the calcium will not be absorbed. And if you can't break down the calcium, your body is robbed of the calcium needed to support bodily functions. Based on the above analysis, I strongly urge you not take the tablet form of calcium. After careful study, I believe that Nutrametrix, blended with Vitamin D_3 and magnesium, isotonic form, supplies the best calcium.

Regular weightbearing exercise. These types of exercises include increased walking, jogging, stair climbing, dancing, Tai chi, and tennis. Muscle-strengthening exercises include weight training and other resistive exercises. Weightbearing exercise programs not only increase bone density, but also improve both muscle strength and the functional ability of the heart and lung.

Other preventive measures. You should avail yourself of all preventive procedures, such as checking and correcting vision and hearing, evaluating any neurological problems, reviewing any prescription medications for side effects that may affect balance, and providing a check list for improving safety at home. Wearing undergarments with hip pad protectors may protect an individual from injuring the hip in the event of a fall. Hip protectors may be considered for those who have significant risk factors for falling or for anyone who has previously fractured a hip.

The avoidance of excessive alcohol intake and tobacco use is very important. Alcohol and cigarettes inhibit osteoblast (cell-building) activities and improve osteoclast (bone-dissolving) cell functioning. Osteoclast cells usually destroy bone density and osteoblast cells build up bone density.

Medical Treatment for Osteoporosis

These are for those with:

- A hip or vertebral fracture.
- A DXA hip or spine T-score that is less or equivalent to −2.5.
- Low bone mass and (U.S. adopted) W.H.O. ten-year probability of hip fractures that are more than,

or equivalent to, 3 percent; or a more than 20 percent ten-year probability of having any major osteoporosis-related fractures.

FDA-approved medications for the treatment of osteoporosis

Bisphosphonates

- Alendronate, brand name, Fosamax. Alendronate reduces the incidence of spine and hip fractures by about 50 percent over three years in people with prior vertebral fractures. It reduces the incidence of vertebral fractures by about 48 percent over three years in those without any prior vertebral fractures.
- Ibandronate, brand name, Boniva. Boniva reduces the incidence of vertebral fractures by about 50 percent over three years.
- Risedronate, brand name, Actonel, with calcium. Risedronate reduces the incidence of vertebral fractures by about 41-plus–49 percent, and nonvertebral fractures by about 36 percent over three years, with a significant reduction of risk occurring after one year of treatment in those with a prior vertebral fracture.
- Zoledronic acid, brand name, Reclast. Zoledronic acid is approved by the FDA, 5mg/IV infusion over at least fifty minutes, once yearly for osteoporosis in postmenopausal women. Reclast reduces the incidence of vertebral fractures by about 70 percent, with significant reduction at one year; it reduces the incidence of hip fractures

by about 41 percent, and of nonvertebral fractures by about 25 percent over three years.

- There are many side effects for bisphosphonates, such as GI problems, difficulty swallowing, inflammation of the esophagus, and gastric ulcer. All these medications must be taken on an empty stomach first thing in the morning with at least eight ounces of plain water.

Other treatments for osteoporosis

- Calcitonin, brand names Miacalcin or Fortical. Oral salmon calcitonin is FDA-approved.
- Estrogen hormone therapy. For estrogen hormone therapy, the Women's Health Initiative reported increased risks of myocardial infarctions, strokes, invasive breast cancer, pulmonary emboli, and deep-vein phlebitis during five years of treatment with conjugated equine estrogen and medroxyprogesterone. Subsequent analysis of those data showed no increase in cardiovascular disease, however, so the use of estrogen hormone treatment is recommended for only a short time in the lowest effective doses. All healthcare providers must evaluate the risks before considering giving their patients this hormonal treatment.
- Parathyroid hormone, PTH, brand name, Forteo. This is approved by the FDA for the treatment of osteoporosis in postmenopausal women at high risk for fracture, although an increased incidence of osteosarcoma in rats has been noted.

Caution is advised in the usage of parathyroid hormone.

TREATMENTS IN TRADITIONAL CHINESE MEDICINE

Traditional Chinese Medicine thinks osteoporosis is mainly caused by kidney deficiency; therefore, the most important thing in TCM is to protect kidney function.

Acupuncture cannot usually treat a fractured bone, but acupuncture can help prevent a broken bone by improving and adjusting the stomach and the small intestine to facilitate their natural absorption of such minerals as calcium, magnesium, and phosphate, and to help prevent the mineral loss that can lead to fractures.

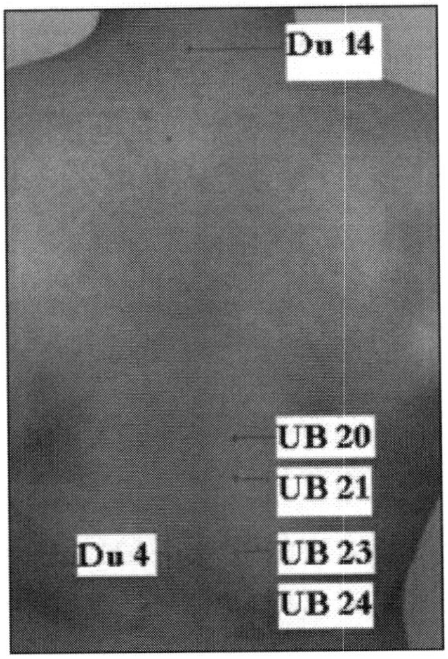

FIGURE 31.1

Acupuncture Points for Osteoporosis

The following acupuncture points are usually selected to help in the prevention of osteoporosis.

- Dazhui Du 14, Ming Men Du 4, Pi Shu UB 20, Wei Shu UB 21, Shen Shu UB 23, and Qi Hai Shu UB 24.

TABLE 31.1

POINTS	MERIDIAN NUMBER	CONDITIONS HELPED
1 Da Zhui	Du 14. See Figure 12.1	See Table 12.2; Figure 12.1
2 Ming Men	Du 4. See Figure 31.1	Stiff back, low back pain, diarrhea, impotence, indigestion, irregular menstruation, nocturnal emissions, vaginal discharge
3 Pi Shu	UB 20. See Figure 31.1	Abdominal pain, abdominal distension, anorexia, back pain, bloody stools, diarrhea, dysentery, swelling, jaundice, profuse menstruation, vomiting
4 Wei Shu	UB 21. See Figure 31.1	Anorexia, chest muscle pain, diarrhea, abdominal pain, rumbling/growling stomach, nausea, vomiting
5 Shen Shu	UB 23. See Figure 31.1	See Table 13.1; Figure 13.1
6 Qi Hai Shu	UB 24. See Figure 31.1	Low back pain, irregular menstruation, asthma

Please refer to the accompanying Figures (illustrations) for the locations of the points. And please note that these illustrations are for information only and may not show all the exact locations of the acupuncture points.

EMILY'S TREATMENT

Emily was treated with above points once a week for 3 months. She was asked to take vitamin D, 800 IU, and 1500mg of calcium per day. In the meantime, she also actively participated in the rehabilitation program in my office and once a day she walks 1.5 miles with a 1.5lb sand bag on each leg. After about three months of therapy, the acupuncture treatments stopped, but she still takes the vitamin D and calcium supplements. After one year, she took the bone density test, which showed that her BMD had started to improve. Emily's successful treatment clearly demonstrates that osteoporosis is a treatable disease, and that there is good chance for women to regain their bone density after the combination treatment of acupuncture, vitamin D, and calcium. Acupuncture helps to improve calcium absorption by the body, as well as strengthen muscles in order to prevent falls.

TIPS TO USE AT HOME OR OFFICE

Lifestyle changes, best started young.

- Make sure to get enough calcium and vitamin D.
- Stop smoking.
- Avoid excessive alcohol intake.
- Engage in weightbearing exercises.
- Recognize any family history of osteoporosis and consult your healthcare provider if there is any family history.

- If you are at high risk for falls, consider using hip protectors, such as Safehip, which will help prevent hip fractures.
- Avoid excessive physical exercise, such as long-term training for bike races, marathons, or similar.

32

Diabetes

CONTROLLING JENNY'S DIABETES MELLITUS

Jenny S. is a fifty-six-year-old woman who was first diagnosed with diabetes mellitus about twenty years ago. She was given insulin injections plus oral anti-diabetes medication, such as metformin, which she took for twenty years and always kept her blood sugar under control. During the past two years, however, she gradually started to feel numbness and a tingling sensation, and sometimes burning pain in both feet, toes, and legs, and sometimes in both arms, hands, and fingers. She also reported a sense of muscle wasting in both the hands and feet, and sometimes dizziness, especially when standing up from a sitting or lying position. She experiences headaches and fainting, and occasionally has poor digestion, even nausea and vomiting. Jenny went to see her primary care physician who checked her blood sugar and A1c levels. Her A1c level was high, but her blood sugar was under good control. However, due to the constant pain, numbness, and tingling sensation, she was referred to me for evaluation and treatment.

I examined her hands and feet and realized that the muscles of the hands and feet had been wasting gradually. She manifested decreased sensation in both her hands and feet. When I used a pin to touch Jenny's feet and hands, she felt burning and an extremely sharp pain sensation. Her feet and hands also felt cold at times. Checking her blood pressure, I found it to be 130/85, slightly above the normal blood pressure of 120/80. Jenny appeared to have orthostatic hypotension, a form of hypotension in which a person's blood pressure suddenly falls when the person stands up—it may be most pronounced after resting.

THE HEMOGLOBIN AIC TEST

The hemoglobin (hb) A1c blood test measures a 2–3 month average of blood sugar. What you eat the night before the HbA1C blood test does NOT affect the result. The test can be done in a lab at any time of day using a sample of blood from your arm.

DEFINITION AND CAUSES OF DIABETES MELLITUS

Diabetes mellitus is a group of a metabolic diseases characterized by high blood-sugar levels. There are two ways that diabetes can occur.

1. When the body cannot produce enough insulin to digest the body's sugar due to defects in insulin secretion, the end result is diabetes.
2. When the insulin receptors in the body are deficient, the result is insulin-resistant diabetes. Located on the cells' surface, normal insulin receptors will accept insulin and trigger the chemical change to digest blood sugar inside the cell, but when they are deficient this does not occur.

If the insulin levels decrease, or if the insulin receptor is defective, the chain of blood-sugar digestion will be damaged. This will cause an increase of blood sugar in the blood, which will, in turn, cause organ damage.

Type 1 Diabetes Mellitus

Type 1 diabetes is characterized by a loss of insulin-producing beta cells in the pancreas, leading to a deficiency of the hormone insulin. Briefly, the beta cells in the pancreas are either defective or fewer in number, so there is not enough insulin produced and the body cannot sufficiently digest blood sugar because of the deficiency of insulin.

When functioning properly, the insulin produced in the pancreas enables the body's cells to absorb glucose and turn it into energy. If the cells do not absorb the glucose, it accumulates in the blood, and leads to vascular, nerve, and other complications.

Although type 1 diabetes is found in some adults, it is most often seen in children, which is why it was formerly called juvenile diabetes.

TESTS FOR DIABETES

If your doctor suspects you have diabetes, he or she will send you for a fasting plasma glucose test (FPG), an oral glucose tolerance test (OGTT) or a Hemoglobin A1C Test (HbA1C). A high blood-sugar reading on any of these tests may mean you have diabetes. To be sure, your doctor will likely repeat the test on another day.

FPG test: For the FPG, you will fast overnight and then have your blood drawn at a lab or doctor's office. A blood sugar reading of:

- 126mg/dL or more likely means you have diabetes.
- 100mg/dL to 125mg/dL may mean you have pre-diabetes.

• 99mg/dL or less means your blood sugar is normal.

OGTT test: You will fast for at least eight hours and then have your blood drawn at a lab. Next, you will drink a sugary beverage and have blood drawn again two hours later. After two hours, a blood glucose reading of:

• 200mg/dL or more may mean you have diabetes.

• 140mg/dL to 199mg/dL likely means you have pre-diabetes.

• 139mg/dL and below means your blood sugar is normal.

HbAlC test: The A1C test is a simple blood test that is usually performed in a lab. You don't need to change your diet or medications before the A1C test. A small sample of blood will be drawn from a vein in your arm.

• 6.5 percent or higher may mean you have diabetes.

• 5.7 to 6.4 percent means you have prediabetes.

Hb A1c is a very good tracking index for the results of treating diabetes. After 90 days of treatment, HbA1c is examined and if HbA1c is less than 7 percent, this is considered good glycemic control. If those with diabetes have HbA1c levels within 7 percent or less than 6.5 percent, they will have significantly lower complications from diabetes, including retinopathy and diabetic neuropathy.

Positive results should be confirmed by a repeat of any of the above methods on a different day.

Type 2 Diabetes Mellitus

Type 2 diabetes is the most common form of diabetes where one of two things can occur: Either the body does not produce enough insulin or the cells ignore the insulin. This latter is known as insulin resistance and is caused by a deficiency or a defect of the insulin receptors in the cell membranes.

In the early stages of type 2 diabetes, the predominant abnormality is reduced insulin sensitivity, characterized by elevated levels of insulin in the blood. At this stage, high blood sugar (hyperglycemia) can be reversed by diet, medications, or a variety of measures that improve insulin sensitivity or reduce glucose production by the liver. As the disease progresses, the impairment of insulin secretion worsens and therapeutic replacement of insulin becomes necessary.

CHRONIC COMPLICATIONS OF DIABETES

Diabetes mainly causes vascular disease. When diabetes is present, the endothelial cells lining the blood vessels take in more glucose than normal since they do not depend on insulin. These cells then form more surface glycoprotein—a sugar (carbohydrate) attached to important integral proteins where they play a role in cell-to-cell interactions—than normal and cause the base membrane to grow thicker and weaker, which results in two main types of vascular disease—microvascular and macrovascular.

Microvascular Diseases

Microvascular diseases include the following.

- **Diabetic cardiomyopathy.** This is damage to the heart, leading to irregular heartbeats and eventually heart failure.
- **Diabetic nephropathy.** High blood sugar damages the endothelial cells of the kidney, and can lead to chronic renal failure, which will eventually require hemodialysis.
- **Diabetic retinopathy.** High blood sugar forms new blood vessels in the retina and macula, and macular edema and will cause severe vision loss or blindness.

DIABETIC NEUROPATHY

In addition to the three microvascular diseases mentioned above, this fourth type most commonly affects people with diabetes, and requires a more detailed discussion.

With this microvascular disease, high blood sugar causes an abnormally decreased sensation, starting with the feet, but potentially occurring in other nerves as well, and often involving fingers and hands at a later stage. This common problem affecting people with diabetes has four distinct types.

Peripheral neuropathy. Peripheral neuropathy, also called distal symmetric neuropathy or sensory motor neuropathy, affects nerves in the arms and legs. Symptoms of peripheral neuropathy may include the following.

- Tingling, burning, or prickling sensation.
- Numbness and sensitivity to pain or temperature.
- Sharp pains or cramps.
- Extreme sensitivity to even a light touch.
- Loss of balance and coordination.
- Muscle weakness and loss of reflexes, especially at the ankle, leading to changes in the way a person walks, and also to feet deformities, such as hammertoes and collapse of the mid foot.
- Because of decreased sensation, people with diabetes can also have skin damage without noticing it, and this can result in skin ulcers. The infection can spread to the bone and the foot may eventually have to be amputated.

Autonomic neuropathy. This mainly affects the nerves that regulate the blood pressure and control the heart and blood glucose levels. Autonomic neuropathy also affects other internal organs, such as the digestive system, respiratory function, urination, sexual response, and vision. The main symptoms are dizziness, fainting, heart palpitations, poor digestion, shortness of breath, urinary incontinency, impotence, or orthostatic hypotension.

Proximal neuropathy. The main symptom of this neuropathy is pain, starting in the thighs, hips, buttocks, or legs, usually on one side of the body. This form is most commonly seen in type 2 diabetes. Proximal neuropathy causes weakness in the legs and the inability to go from a sitting to a standing position without help.

Focal neuropathy. Focal neuropathy usually affects a few specific nerves. Most commonly, the person is unable to focus the eye, has double vision, aching behind one eye, or paralysis, such as Bell's Palsy, on one side of the face, severe pain in the lower back or pelvis, pain in the front of the thigh, the chest, the stomach, or the side.

Treatment of Diabetic Neuropathy

The most important treatment involves lowering the blood sugar to a normal range to prevent further nerve damage. Since pain is the main symptom of diabetic neuropathy, pain relief is the second most important treatment after controlling the blood sugar.

Macrovascular Diseases

When blood sugar is deposited in the medial and large blood vessels, it will cause atherosclerosis. There are five types of macrovascular disease.

- Coronary artery disease, which will lead to angina and myocardial infarction.
- Strokes. The blood vessels supplying the brain tissue are blocked, leading to brain tissue damage and paralysis of the opposite side of the face and body.
- Peripheral vascular disease, which will cause intermittent claudication and difficulty walking.
- Diabetic myonecrosis, which will cause muscle wasting of the four extremities.
- Carotid artery stenosis. This will cause dizziness, fainting, and sometimes a stroke.

TREATMENTS IN WESTERN MEDICINE

The main goal in the treatment of diabetes is to strictly control or minimize any elevation of blood sugar without abnormally lowering its levels.

- **Type 1 diabetes** is treated with insulin, exercise, and a specific diabetes diet.

- **Type 2 diabetes** is treated first with weight reduction, a diabetes diet, and exercise. If these treatments fail to control the elevated blood sugar, oral medications, such as metformin, glyburide, and others are used. If oral medications are still insufficient, insulin is considered.

Pain Medications Used in Western Medicine

Western medicine will control the pain of diabetes with the following medications.

- Tricyclic antidepressants, including amitriptyline, imipramine, or desipramine.
- Celexa, Cymbalta, Paxil, and Wellbutrin can also be used.
- Anticonvulsants, including Lyrica, gabapentin, Neurontin, carbamazepine, or lamotrigine.
- Opioids and opioid-like drugs, such as controlled-release OxyContin, tramadol, or Ultram.

TREATMENTS IN TRADITIONAL CHINESE MEDICINE

Depending on the symptoms, Chinese medicine will treat different symptoms with different groups of acupuncture points. However, it is necessary to remember that acupuncture alone may not lower blood sugar and will not cure the diabetes mellitus. Acupuncture only can modify the symptoms.

For the relief of pain, numbness, and the tingling sensation, there are two groups of acupuncture points that can be used.

Pain Relief for Upper Extremities

TABLE 32.1

POINTS	MERIDIAN NUMBER.	CONDITIONS HELPED
1 Bai Hui	Du 20. See Figure 22.3	See Table 22.4
2 Qu Qi	LI 11. See Figure 12.2	See Table 12.2
3 Zu San Li	St 36. See Figure 13.4	See Table 13.3
4 Wai Guan	Si 5. See Figure 12.3	See Table 12.2
5 He Gu	LI 4. See Figure 12.3	See Table 12.1
6 Ba Xie	Extraordinary Points. See Figure 32.1	Excessive heat, finger numbness, spasms and contractures of the fingers, redness and swelling on the back of the hand

Please refer to the accompanying Figures (illustrations) for the locations of the points. And please note that these illustrations are for information only and may not show all the exact locations of the acupuncture points.

- Du 20 Bai Hui, LI 11 Qu Qi, St 36 Zu San Li, SJ 5 Wai Guan, LI 4 He Gu, and extra points Ba Xie.

Pain Relief for Lower Extremities

- Du 20 Bai Hui, GB 34 Yang Ling Quan, Sp 9 Ying Ling Quan, GB 40 Qiu Xu, GB 41 Zu Ling Qi, UB 64 Jing Gu, and Extra points Ba Feng.

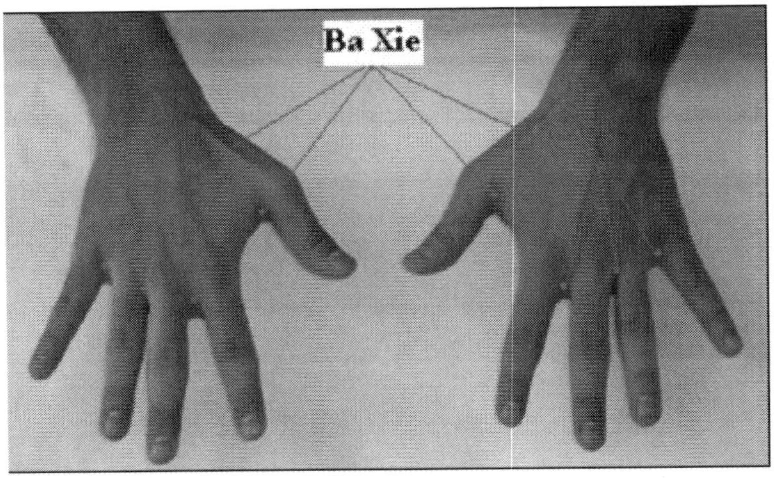

FIGURE 32.1

TABLE 32.2

POINTS	MERIDIAN NUMBER	CONDITIONS HELPED
1 Bai Hui	Du 20. See Figure 22.3	See Table 22.4
2 Yang Ling Quan	GB 34. See Figure 1 S.3	See Table 15.3
3 Ying Ling Quan	Sp 9. See Figure 28.2	See Table 28.1
4 Qiu Xu	GB 40. See Figure 32.2	Pain in the neck, swelling in the armpit region, vomit-ing, acid reflux, muscular atrophy of the lower limbs, pain and swelling of the external ankle bone, malaria

POINTS	MERIDIAN NUMBER	CONDITIONS HELPED
5 Zu Ling Qi	GB 41. See Figure 32.2	Headaches, vertigo, outer eyelid pain, breast pain, irregular menstruation, pain and swelling of the back of the foot, pain spasms of the foot and toe
6 ling Gu	UB 64. See Figure 32.2	Headaches, neck rigidity, pain in the lower back and thigh, epilepsy
7 Ba Feng	Extraordinary points. See Figure 32.2	Toe pain, redness and swelling of the back of the foot

Please refer to the accompanying Figures (illustrations) for the locations of the points. And please note that these illustrations are for information only and may not show all the exact locations of the acupuncture points.

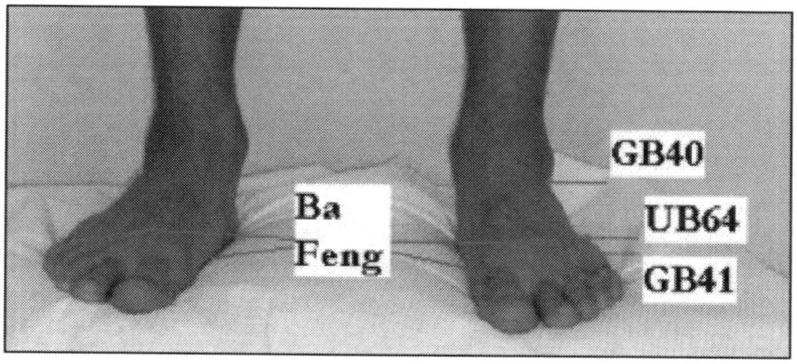

FIGURE 32.2

For Gastrointestinal Problems

If you encounter indigestion, belching, nausea, vomiting, or other GI conditions, the following points should be used.

- Ren 12 Zhong Wan, PC 6 Nei Guan, St 36 Zu San Li, and Sp 9 Ying Ling Quan.

TABLE 32.3

POINTS	MERIDIAN NUMBER	CONDITIONS HELPED
1 Zhong \Van	Ren 12. See Figure 13.3	See Table 13.3
2 Nei Guan	PC 6. See Figure 16.6	See Table 16.1
3 Zu San Li	St 36. See Figure 13.4	See Table 13.3
4 Ying Ling Quan	Sp 9. See Figure 28.2	See Table 28.1

Please refer to the accompanying Figures (illustrations) for the locations of the points. And please note that these illustrations are for information only and may not show all the exact locations of the acupuncture points.

For Dizziness and Weakness

When feeling dizzy while in a sitting or standing position, or because blood pressure drops when standing up from a sitting position, the acupuncture points used should be the following.

- Du 20 Bai Hui, UB 23 Shen Shu, Ki 3 Tai Xi, GB 20 Feng Chi, and Du 24 Shen Ting.

TABLE 32.4

POINTS	MERIDIAN NUMBER	CONDITIONS HELPED
1 Bai Hui	Du 20. See Figure 22.3	See Table 22.4
2 Shen Shu	UB 23. See Figure 14.1	See Table 14.4
3 Tai Xi	Ki 3. See Figure 16.7	See Table 16.2
4 Feng Chi	GB 20. See Figure 12.1	See Table 12.1

POINTS	MERIDIAN NUMBER	CONDITIONS HELPED
5 Shen Ting	Du 24. See Figure 32.3	Anxiety, epilepsy, headaches, insomnia, palpitation, congested or runny nose, vertigo

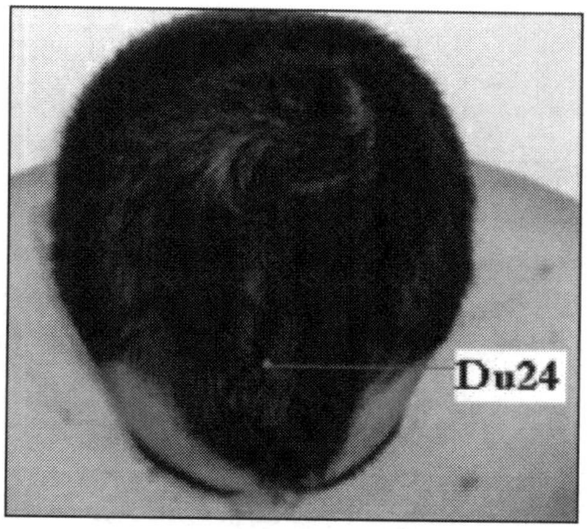

FIGURE 32.3

For Urinary Incontinence and Frequent Infection

Chinese medicine thinks this is a kidney yang deficiency, therefore the following points are used to improve the kidney yang.

- Sp 6 San Ying Jiao, Ren 4 Guan Yuan, Ren 3 Zhong Ji, UB 23 Shen Shu, UB 28 Pang Guang shu, Ki 3 Tai Xi, Ren 6 Qi Hai, and Lu 9 Tai Yuan.

TABLE 32.5

POINTS	MERIDIAN NUMBER	CONDITIONS HELPED
1 San Yin Jiao	Sp 6. See Figure 16.6	See Table 16.1

POINTS	MERIDIAN NUMBER	CONDITIONS HELPED
2 Guan Yuan	Ren 4. See Figure 30.1	See Table 30.1
3 Zhong Ji	Ren 3. See Figure 30.1	See Table 30.1
4 Shen Shu	UB 23. See Figure 14.1	See Table 14.4
5 Pang Guan Shu	UB 28. See Figure 32.5	Retention of urine, incontinence, frequent urination, diarrhea, constipation, stiffness and pain of the lower back
6 Tai Xi	Ki 3. See Figure 16.7	See Table 16.2
7 Qi Hai	Ren 6. See Figure 19.2	See Table 19.3
8 Tai Yuan	Lu 9. See Figure 32.4	Cough, asthma, coughing up blood, sore throat, palpitation, pain in the chest, wrist, and arm

Please refer to the accompanying Figures (illustrations) for the locations of the points. And please note that these illustrations are for information only and may not show all the exact locations of the acupuncture points.

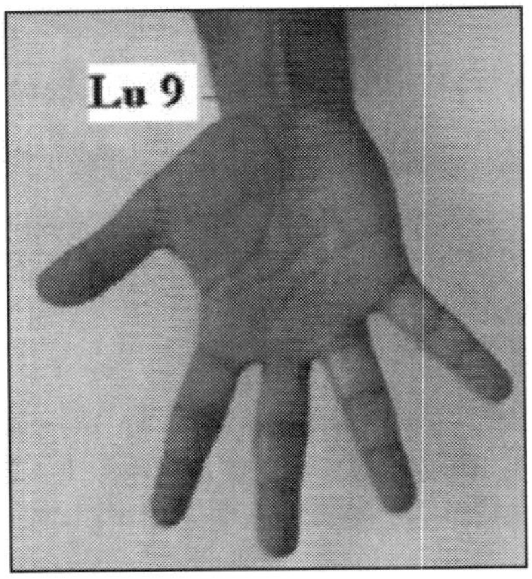

FIGURE 32.4

For Impotence, Decreased Arousal, and Orgasm

- The acupuncture points will be Ren 4 Guan Yuan, Du 4 Min Meng, UB 23 Sheng Shu, Ki 3 Tai Xi, Sp 6 San Ying Jiao, Ren 3 Zhong Ji, UB 20 Pi Shu, and St 36 Zu San Li.

TABLE 32.6

POINTS	MERIDIAN NUMBER	CONDITIONS HELPED
1 Guan Yuan	Ren 4. See Figure 30.1	See Table 30.1
2 Min Men	Du 4. See Figure 31.1	See Table 31.1
3 Shen Shu	UB 23. See Figure 14.1	See Table 14.4
4 Tai Xi	Ki 3. See Figure 16.7	See Table 16.2
5 San Yin Jiao	Sp 6. See Figure 16.6	See Table 16.1
6 Zhong Ji	Ren 3. See Figure 30.1	See Table 30.1
7 Pi Shu	UB 20. See Figure 15.4	See Table 1 S.2
8 Zu San Li	St 36. See Figure 16.4	See Table 13.3

Please refer to the accompanying Figures (illustrations) for the locations of the points. And please note that these illustrations are for information only and may not show all the exact locations of the acupuncture points.

JENNY'S TREATMENT

Even though her blood sugar had been under good control for twenty years, Jenny developed one of the typical chronic complications of diabetes—diabetic neuropathy. With neuropathy in both legs, she felt numbness, tingling, and decreased sensation in both feet—she reported feeling as though she was stepping on cotton as she walked.

I chose the above-mentioned points for lower extremities, plus a special method, blossom needles. Blossom needles are a group of about seven small needles encased in a small plastic hammer that is used to tap the skin and stimulate the nerves on it and underneath it. On each of her twenty visits for both body acupuncture and blossom needles, I used the blossom needles to tap the entire length of her feet and lower legs for approximately twenty minutes. The peripheral neuropathy in her legs is now much improved. As she began to feel her legs more, her gait improved significantly, and she is again able to feel hot water, temperature, and other objects.

Tanks to acupuncture treatments, I was able to successfully diminish the related problems that arose with this neuropathy.

TIPS FOR PEOPLE WITH DIABETES

- The most important thing is to control your blood sugar.
- The pain and numbness of diabetic neuropathy is very difficult to treat, but you can expect that the pain will be brought under control sooner than the numbness and tingling sensation.

33

Hypertension

WILLIAM'S HYPERTENSION LEADS TO A STROKE

William S., a sixty-two-year-old man, works as a stock analyst. His day begins at 6AM and finishes at 7PM. His lifestyle is very stressful, but he is a regular exerciser, running five miles on Saturday and Sunday. He has no health problems, save that he smokes about half a pack of cigarettes a day and has been drinking coffee for thirty years. One morning, on awakening, he felt a sudden onset of weakness and numbness on the left side of his face and arm, as well as in his left leg, and he had a moderate headache. He had difficulty walking and called his wife who noted his speech was slurred. She called an ambulance and he was rushed to the emergency room where his blood pressure was found to be 160/100. A CT scan showed blood in his brain, so William was diagnosed with a hypertensive hemorrhagic stroke. He had emergency open-scalp surgery and the blood clot was removed from his brain, but after the surgery he felt the left side of his face drooping and there was weakness in his left arm and leg.

After three months of intensive physical therapy, his symptoms improved, but he asked his doctor how, considering that he eats right and exercises, he could have suffered a stroke. He did mention to the doctor that he had not been checked for hypertension for five years, though he and his wife had availed themselves of the free blood-pressure monitor at their local supermarket.

The doctor put him on two different antihypertensive medications and told him he needed to have his blood pressure checked yearly by his physician. For a correct blood pressure reading, the doctor advised him that the readings should be taken three times, at least a week apart, and then the numbers should be averaged.

HYPERTENSION—A LEADING CAUSE OF STROKES

Hypertension is high blood pressure and it is one of the main causes of a stroke. A person can have high blood pressure for years without knowing it because high blood pressure usually has no symptoms, though occasionally headaches may occur. During this asymptomatic period, hypertension can do damage to multiple organs, such as the heart, the blood vessels, the kidneys, or the brain. For this reason, it is referred to as a silent killer because suddenly one day the hypertensive person has a stroke, or develops coronary heart disease or kidney failure.

The following comprise the rule of thumb on how to accurately and effectively take blood pressure.

- Blood pressure should be taken at least one hour after caffeine, thirty minutes after smoking or strenuous exercise, and without any stress present.
- The person should be upright in a chair with both feet flat on the floor for a minimum of five minutes prior to taking a reading.
- Some people feel nervous on seeing doctors, a fairly common phenomenon known as white coat syndrome. To avoid this, the person getting the reading should be in a relaxed situation in an isolated room. Also, to counteract any discrepancy and assure an accurate result, three blood pressure readings should be taken at least five minutes apart and the results should then be averaged.
- Older people who are suspected of having orthostatic hypotension should be given initial measurements in both arms. And in order to obtain the correct blood pressure readings, this should be done in lying, sitting, and standing blood positions.

DEFINITION OF HYPERTENSION (HTN)

Based on the U.S. National Heart, Lung, and Blood Institute 2003 guidelines, blood pressure is defined as follows.

- For adults age eighteen and above, normal systolic blood pressure is less than 120mmHg, and diastolic blood pressure is less than 80mmHg.

- Pre-hypertension systolic is 120–139, with diastolic is between 80–89.
- Stage 1 hypertension is between 140–159 systolic, with diastolic between 90 and more than 99.
- Stage 2 hypertension is more than 160 systolic, with diastolic more than 100.

TABLE 33.1. CLASSIFICATION OF BLOOD PRESSURE (BP) FOR ADULTS

BP CLASSIFICATION	SYSTOLIC BP MMHG	DIASTOLIC BP MMHG	LIFESTYLE MODIFICATION
Normal	< 120	< 80	Encourage
Prehypertension	120–139	80–89	Yes
Stage 1 HTN	140–159	90–99	Yes
Stage 2 HTN	> or=160	> or=100	Yes

Sources: 7th Report of the Joint National Committee on the Prevention, Detection, Evaluation, and Treatment of High Blood Pressure (JNC 7), 2003

THE TWO MAJOR FORMS OF HYPERTENSION

Essential or Primary Hypertension

Ninety-five percent of those with hypertension exhibit essential or primary symptoms. Essential hypertension indicates that either no specific medical cause can be found to explain the person's condition or that it might be caused by multiple factors. Those combined effects are responsible for HTN in approximately 72 million Americans.

Secondary Hypertension

This accounts for 5 percent of those with hypertension. In this instance, the high blood pressure is secondary to a specific abnormality, as for example kidney disease or tumors, adrenal adenoma, or other endocrine tumors.

IDENTIFIABLE CAUSES OF HYPERTENSION

- Sleep apnea
- Drug induced (or related) causes
- Chronic kidney diseases
- Primary aldosteronism (adrenal gland overproduction of the hormone aldosterone)
- Renovascular disease
- Chronic steroid treatment
- Cushing's syndrome (hormone disorder caused by high level of cortisol in blood)
- Adrenal gland tumor (pheochromocytoma)
- Narrowing (coarctation) of the aorta
- Thyroid or parathyroid disease

HOW WESTERN MEDICINE INVESTIGATES NEWLY DIAGNOSED HYPERTENSION

A physician will try to identify possible causes of secondary hypertension and seek evidence of end-organ damage to the heart, eyes, or kidneys.

Damages to Target Organs—Heart

- Muscle thickening (hypertrophy) in left ventricle, the heart's main pumping chamber
- Angina or prior myocardial infarction
- Heart failure

Damages to Other Target Organs

- The brain: A stroke or a transient ischemic attack
- The kidneys: Chronic kidney disease
- The arteries: Peripheral artery disease
- The eyes: Damage to the retina of the eye (retinopathy)

MAIN BLOOD TESTS PERFORMED TO DETERMINE CAUSES AND RESULTS OF HTN

Renal function. Creatinine test to identify any underlying renal disease as a cause of hypertension, as well as it causing the onset of kidney damage.

In the meantime, a baseline needs to be set up to monitor the possible side effects of certain antihypertensive drugs on the kidneys.

Electrolytes, including sodium, potassium, calcium, chloride.

Glucose to identify diabetes mellitus.

Cholesterol to identify the possible cause of coronary artery disease.

Urine samples. A healthcare provider might take urine samples to check for proteinuria in order to find out if there is any underlying kidney disease or evidence of hypertensive renal damage.

EKG for evidence of any damage to the heart.

Chest x-ray to check for signs of cardiac enlargement.

A recent survey found that 30 percent of those with hypertension were not aware they had it; 41 percent did not receive any antihypertensive treatment; and only 34 percent of those surveyed had it under proper control.

PREVENTION OF HYPERTENSION

Prevention of damage related to high blood pressure is the most important issue, and lowering blood pressure to prevent end-organ damage to the retina, kidney, heart, or brain is crucial. The following prevention procedures are recommended by National Institute of Health and W.H.O.

- Weight reduction and regular aerobic exercise, such as walking, running, swimming, or bicycling. Several studies indicated that lower-intensity exercise may be more effective in lowering blood pressure than higher-intensity exercise.
- Reducing sodium in the diet decreases blood pressure in about 33 percent of people.
- Reducing sugar intake also helps.
- Quitting smoking and decreasing alcohol consumption to a minimum.
- Adopting the DASH (Dietary Approaches to Stop Hypertension) eating plan, which is rich in potassium and calcium, with reduced dietary sodium.

Lifestyle Modifications

Modifying lifestyles can reduce blood pressure, enhance antihypertensive efficacy, and decrease cardiovascular risk. As an example, a 1600mg sodium eating plan has effects similar to single drug therapy. Combinations of two or more lifestyle modifications can achieve even better results.

TABLE 33.2. THE BENEFITS OF LIFESTYLE MODIFICATIONS IN MANAGING HYPERTENSION

MODIFICATION	RECOMMENDATION	BENEFITS
Weight reduction	Maintain normal body weight (mass index 18.S–24.9)	If you can lose 10Kg, you may be able to lower your blood pressure about 5–20mmHg

MODIFICATION	RECOMMENDATION	BENEFITS
Adopt DASH eating plan	Consume a diet rich in fruits, vegetables, and low–fat dairy products with a reduced content of saturated and total fat	If you adopt this plan, you may be able to lower your blood pressure about 8–14mmHg
Dietary sodium reduction	Reduce dietary sodium intake to no more than 100mmol per day (2.4g sodium or 6g sodium chloride)	If you adopt this modification in your diet, you may be able to lower your blood pressure about 4–9mmHg
Physical activity	Engage in regular aerobic physical activity, such as brisk walking at least thirty minutes per day most days of the week	If you adopt this plan, you may be able to lower your blood pressure about 2–4mmHg
Moderation of alcohol consumption	Limit consumption to no more than 2 drinks (1oz or 30ml ethanol, 24oz beer, 10oz wine, or 3oz 80 proof whiskey) per day in most men, and to no more than 1 drink per day in women and lighter weight people	If you adopt this modification, you may be able to lower your blood pressure about 2–4mmHg

Sources: 7th Report of the Joint National Committee on the Prevention, Detection, Evaluation, and Treatment of High Blood Pressure (JNC 7), 2003

PHARMACEUTICAL TREATMENT OF HYPERTENSION

There are many people who are currently using pharmaceutical drugs, such as angiotensin-converting enzyme inhibitors (ACE inhibitors), angiotensin receptor blockers (ARBs), beta-blockers, calcium channel blockers, and thiazide type diuretics.

Diuretics of the thiazide type have been the basis of antihypertensive therapy in most outcome trials. In many studies, a diuretic works much better than other antihypertensive medications. Therefore, in the United States, the thiazide-type diuretic is the first choice to treat hypertension.

TABLE 33.3. COMMONLY USED DRUGS

CLASS	NAME (TRADE NAME)	USUAL DOSE RANGE IN MG/DAY	USUAL DAILY FREQUENCY
Thiazide diuretics	Chlorothiazide (Diuril)	125–500	1–2
Loop diuretics	Furosemide (Lasix)	20–80	2
Potassium–sparing diuretics	Amiloride (Midamor); Triamterene (Dyrenium)	5–10; 50–100	1–2; 1–2
Aldosterone receptor blockers	Spironolactone (Aldactone)	25–50	1
Angiotensin converting enzyme inhibitors	Lisinopril (Prinivil, Zestrilt); Quinapril (Accupril)	10–40; 10–80	1; 1
Angiotensin II antagonists	Irbesartan (Avapro); Losartan (Cozaar)	150–300; 25–100	1; 1–2
Beta–blockers	Atenolol (Tenormin)	25–00	1
Calcium channel blockers: Dihydropyridines	Amlodipine (Norvasc)	2.5–10	1
Calcium channel blockers: non–Dihydropyridines	Diltiazem extended release	180–420	1

Sources: 7th Report of the Joint National Committee on the Prevention, Detection, Evaluation, and Treatment of High Blood Pressure (JNC 7), 2003.

Thiazide-type diuretics should be used alone or in combination with one of the other classes, such ACE inhibitors, angiotensin receptor blockers, beta-blockers, or calcium channel blockers.

The Goal of Antihypertensive Therapy

The ultimate public health goal of antihypertensive therapy is the reduction of high blood pressure and cardiovascular disease. The aim of treatment for most people should be getting blood pressure readings to <140/90mmHg, and even lower in certain contexts, such as diabetes or kidney disease (some medical professionals recommend keeping levels below 120/80mmHg).

Achieving Blood-Pressure Control

Most people who are hypertensive will require two or more antihypertensive medications to achieve their blood-pressure goals. An additional second drug from a different class should be initiated when the use of a single drug in inadequate doses fails to achieve the blood-pressure goal. When the blood pressure is more than 20/10mmHg above the goal, consideration should be given to initiate therapy with two drugs, either as separate prescriptions or in fixed dose combinations. However, the likelihood of a dramatic decline in blood pressure leading to dizziness when people attempt to stand (orthostatic hypotension), must be mentioned, as it can occur in people who have diabetes, or in older people and there could be a dysfunction of the autonomic nervous system that regulates unconscious body functions, including blood pressure and heart rates.

TREATMENT FOR HYPERTENSION IN TRADITIONAL CHINESE MEDICINE—ACUPUNCTURE

There is a thousand year history of acupuncture treatment for different symptoms of hypertension, but there is no word in Chinese history for *hypertension.* The hypertension diagnosis is always found where there are symptoms of dizziness, faintness, strokes, and headaches. In recent studies, it was shown that acupuncture treatment can be an excellent adjunct to medical treatment, especially for those who are diagnosed with prehypertension or stage 1 hypertension, even stage 2 hypertension. In these instances, acupuncture might greatly decrease the dosage of antihypertensive medications, and also decrease the side effects of these medications. I do not, however, recommend discontinuing antihypertensive medications and using acupuncture as the only treatment.

In traditional Chinese medicine, hypertension is manifested as following two types.

Excessive Liver Yang

The person usually shows dizziness, tinnitus, and headaches, sometimes emotional upset, anger, facial redness, insomnia, and vivid dreams or nightmares. The treatment should be focused on lowering the excessive liver yang.

- The points should be liver UB 18 Gan Shu, Liv 3 Tai Chong, GB 43 Xia Xi, UB 23 Shen Shu, GB 20 Feng Chi, Li 4 He Gu, and Li 11 Qu Qi.
- Sp 6 San Yin Jiao, PC 6 Nei Guan, and GB 41 Zu Ling Qi are sometimes added.

TABLE 33.4

POINTS	MERIDIAN NUMBER	CONDITIONS HELPED
I Can Shu	UB 18. See Figure 19.1	See Table 19.3
2 Tai Chong	Liv 3. See Figure 15.3	See Table 15.3
3 Xia Xi	GB 43. See Figure 33.1	Headaches, dizziness and vertigo, tinnitus, deafness, swelling of the cheek, pain in the breast, fever
4 Shen Shu	UB 23. See Figure 14.1	See Table 14.4
5 Feng Chi	Gallbladder 20. See Figure 22.4	See Table 22.1
6 He Gu	Li 4. See Figure 12.3	See Table 22.2
7 Qu Qi	Li 11. See Figure 12.2	See Table 12.2

POINTS	MERIDIAN NUMBER	CONDITIONS HELPED
8 San Yin Jiao	Sp 6. See Figure 16.6	See Table 16.1
9 Nei Guan	PC 6. See Figure 16.7	See Table 16.1
10 Zu Ling Qi	GB 41. See Figure 33.1	Headaches, vertigo, pain in the breast, irregular menstruation, pain and swelling of the back of the foot, spastic pain of the foot and toe

Please refer to the accompanying Figures (illustrations) for the locations of the points. And please note that these illustrations are for information only and may not show all the exact locations of the acupuncture points.

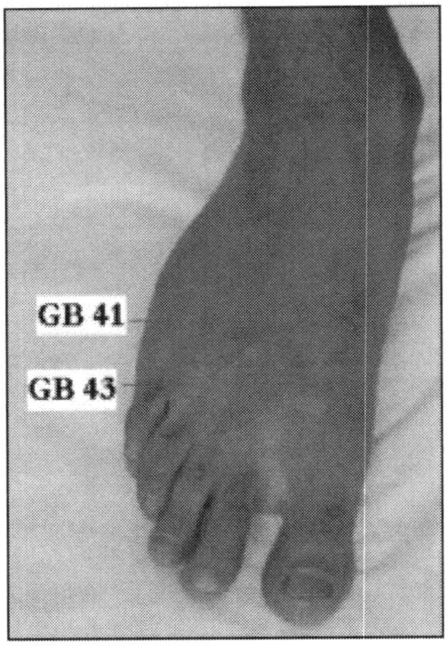

FIGURE 33.1

Deficiency of Blood and Qi (Energy)

The person very often feels dizziness and faintness; the dizziness is triggered by fatigue and always becomes worse when getting up from a sitting position. This deficiency is always accompanied by a pale face, and sometimes heart palpitations, insomnia, fatigue, slowed speech, and poor appetite. The treatment for this condition should be focused on nourishing the qi and blood and improving the function of the spleen and stomach. The acupuncture points for this are the following.

- UB 20 Pi Shu, St 36 Zu San Li, Du 20 Bai Hui, Ren 6 Qi Hai, Li 3 Zhang Men, Du 24 Shen Ting, and Li 4 He Gu.
- For an acute hypertensive crisis, Extra Point Tai Yang, Du 20 Bai Hui, and St 40 Fen Long can be used.
- Some studies show that by piercing extra points of Tai Yang and Yin Tang with slight bleeding the blood pressure will usually drop quickly.
- If there is a severe headache in the forehead, UB 2 Zan Zhu is used.
- If the headache is on the top of scalp, Du 20 Bai Hui and Extra Point Si Shen Chong are added.
- If there is neck pain with stiffness, GB 20 Feng Chi is used.
- If there is dizziness accompanied with tinnitus, St 8 Tou Wei is also added.

TABLE 33.5

POINTS	MERIDIAN NUMBER	CONDITIONS HELPED
1 Pi Shu	UB 20. See Figure 15.4	See Table 15.2
2 Zu San Li	St 36. See Figure 13.4	See Table 13.3

POINTS	MERIDIAN NUMBER	CONDITIONS HELPED
3 Bai Hui	Du 20. See Figure 22.3	See Table 22.4
4 Qi Hai	Ren 6. See Figure 14.2	See Table 14.4
5 Zhang Men	Li 3. See Figure 18.4	See Table 18.1
6 Shen Ting	Du 24. See Figure 33.2	Anxiety, epilepsy, headaches, insomnia, palpitations, runny nose, vertigo
7 Feng Long	St 40. See Figure 13.4	See Table 13.3
8 Tai Yang	Extra Point. See Figure 22.2	See Table 22.2
9 Yin Tang	Extra Point. See Figure 22.1	See Table 22.2
10 Zan Zhu	UB 2. See Figure 15.1	See Table 15.1
11 Si Shen Chong	Extra–HN 1. See Figure 17.2	See Table 17.2
12 Feng Chi	GB 20. See Figure 12.1	See Table 12.1
13 Tou Wei	St 8. See Figure 22.5	See Table 22.3

Please refer to the accompanying Figures (illustrations) for the locations of the points. And please note that these illustrations are for information only and may not show all the exact locations of the acupuncture points.

TREATMENT FOR WILLIAM

William was diagnosed with excessive liver yang and underwent my treatment. After three months, his blood pressure became stable and under control, and only minimum dosages of the antihypertensive drugs were used.

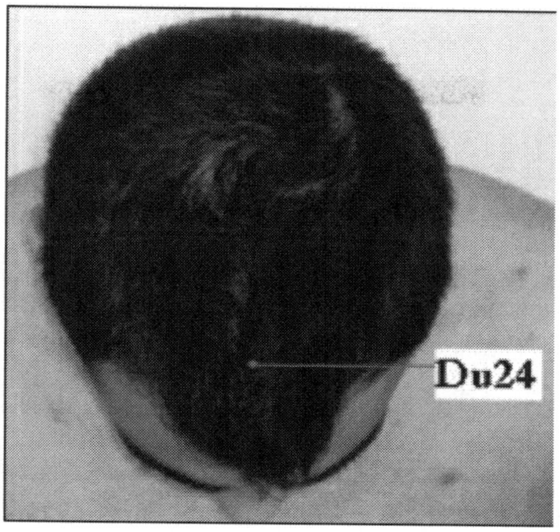

FIGURE 33.2

TIPS TO USE AT HOME OR OFFICE

- Be calm and relaxed. Do not add stress on top of your blood pressure.
- Massaging Tai Yang and Bai Hui will usually help you decrease your headache and your blood pressure. Acupressure the points with your thumb or knuckle, pressing with comfortable pressure on the points; count to 20, then change to another point.
- After the blood pressure comes down, maintenance with acupuncture is necessary once a week in the short term, and is also very useful and effective in the long run.

34

Chemotherapy Symptoms

ALLEVIATING AMANDA'S CHEMOTHERAPY SYMPTOMS

Amanda W. is a forty-five-year-old woman who was diagnosed two years ago with stage 3A cancer symptoms in her left breast. She was screened by a mammogram and an ultrasound, which found a tumor about one inch across on her left breast, with five positive lymph nodes under her left arm. She had a mastectomy on the left side, with clearance of the lymph nodes under the left arm. She also was given chemotherapy for about three months. After chemotherapy, Amanda complained of nausea, vomiting, diarrhea, and a change of taste in her mouth; she also felt very weak and fatigued. She experienced hair loss and poor concentration, with occasional numbness and tingling on the tips of her finger and toes, and came to me for help in relieving or decreasing these multiple side effects of her chemotherapy.

BREAST CANCER STATISTICS

In the United States, breast cancer is the second most common type of cancer among women. And among women worldwide, after non-melanoma skin cancer, breast cancer is the most common form of cancer. It is the number-one cause of cancer death in Hispanic women, and is the second most common cause of cancer death in white, black, Asian/Pacific Islander, and American Indian/Alaska Native women.

In 2005 (the most recent year numbers are available):

- 186,467 women and 1,764 men were diagnosed with breast cancer;[1][2]
- 41,116 women and 375 men died from breast cancer.[1][2]

RISK FACTORS FOR BREAST CANCER

The key to preventing breast cancer is knowing the risk factors and practicing self-screening. The following risk factors might increase your chances of developing breast cancer:

- Age. The older you are, the higher the chance that you can develop breast cancer. In women over sixty, there is usually a higher chance of breast cancer than in women under sixty.
- A previous history of breast cancer.
- Family history. If a mother, sister, or daughter had breast cancer, or if breast cancer runs anywhere in your family, the risk is higher than for the average woman.

- Gene changes. If you have the BRCA1or BRCA2 genes, you will probably have a higher chance of developing breast cancer.
- Reproductive history. The older a woman is when she had her first child, the greater her chances of developing breast cancer will be.
- Women without children are at increased risk of breast cancer.
- If you got your first menstrual period before age twelve, there is an increased risk for breast cancer.
- If you became menopausal after age fifty-five, there is an increased risk of breast cancer.
- Menopausal women using hormone therapy with estrogen plus and progestin after menopause are at increased risk of breast cancer.
- Race. White women have a higher chance of developing breast cancer than darker-skinned women.
- Breast density. The higher the density of breast tissue, the higher the chance of breast cancer.
- Overweight or obese women have a higher chance of breast cancer.
- Lack of physical activity leads to a higher chance of breast cancer.
- Alcohol consumption in immoderate amounts leads to a higher chance of breast cancer.

SCREENING MAMMOGRAMS

A mammogram is a picture of the breast made with x-rays. The National Cancer Institute recommends the following:

- Women in their forties and older should have a mammogram every one to two years.
- Women who are younger than forty and who have risk factors for breast cancer should ask their healthcare provider whether to have mammograms and how often to have them.

If a mammogram is positive, the following procedures might be recommended.

- Ultrasound. This will identify if the lump is a fluid-filled cyst or a solid mass.
- MRI. This will give a detailed picture of the breast tissue.
- Needle biopsy, core biopsy, and surgical biopsy.

STAGES OF BREAST CANCER

Here are the stages of breast cancer.

- Stage 0 is carcinoma in situ. Abnormal cells are in the lining of a lobule or in the lining of a duct.
- Stage 1 is 2cm or smaller and has not spread outside the breast.
- Stage 2 is one of the following: The tumor is no more than 5cm, with or without it spreading to the lymph nodes under the arm.

- Stage 3 is locally advanced cancer. It is divided into stages 3A, 3B, and 3C.

CANCER STATISTICS

According to the *United States Cancer Statistics 2005* from the Centers for Disease Control and Prevention, the following statistical data showed the chances of cancer for American men and women. (The numbers in parentheses are the age-adjusted—U.S. standard—rates per 100,000 people.) www.cdc.gov/Featu res/CancerStatistics/

Cancer Among Men

The three most common cancers among men include:

- Prostate cancer (142.4): First among men of all races.
- Lung cancer (84.6): Second among men of all races.
- Colorectal cancer (58.2): Third among men of all races.

The leading causes of cancer death among men are:

- Lung cancer (69.4): First among men of all races.
- Prostate cancer (25.4): Second among white (22.7), black (54.1), American Indian/Alaska Native (18.0), and Hispanic (18.7) men.
- Liver cancer: Second among Asian/Pacific Islander men (14.5).

- Colorectal cancer (21.0): Third among men of all races.

Cancer Among Women

The three most common cancers among women include:

- Breast cancer (117.7): First among women of all races.
- Lung cancer (55.2): Second among white (56.6), black (50.9), and American Indian/Alaska Native (37.6) women, and third among Asian/Pacific Islander (26.9) and Hispanic (25.2) women.
- Colorectal cancer (41.9): Second among Asian/Pacific Islander (32.2) and Hispanic (33.9) women, and third among white (40.8), black (49.4), and American Indian/Alaska Native women (24.5).

The leading causes of cancer death among women are:

- Lung cancer (40.6): First among white (41.6), black (40.2), Asian/Pacific Islander (18.2), and American Indian/Alaska Native (29.2) women, and second among Hispanic women (14.4).
- Breast cancer (24.0): First among Hispanic women (15.1), and second among white (23.3), black (32.9), Asian/Pacific Islander (12.3), and American Indian/Alaska Native (15.3) women.
- Colorectal cancer (14.6): Third among women of all races.

Racial or Ethnic Variations

- American Indian/Alaska Native men have the lowest incidence rates of cancer; however, Asian/Pacific Islander men have the lowest death rates from cancer.
- White women have the highest incidence rates of cancer; however, black women have the highest death rates from cancer.
- American Indian/Alaska Native women have the lowest incidence rates of cancer and the third-highest death rates from cancer.

SIDE EFFECTS OF CHEMOTHERAPY

Many cancers are treated with chemotherapy IV in their various stages. Therefore, different side effects will accompany the chemotherapy. The main organ or tissues of the human body that may be affected by chemotherapy doses are where normal cells rapidly divide and grow, such as the lining of the mouth, the digestive system, skin, hair, and bone marrow. After a treatment period longer than six months, your nervous system will be affected as well, and the symptoms of this, including poor concentration, decreased memory, peripheral polyneuropathy, and tinnitus, might appear. Long-term side effects can also include weight gain, loss of fertility, menopause, and secondary cancer, such as leukemia.

Short-Term Side Effects

- In the digestive system, some chemotherapy drugs can cause nausea and vomiting, even diarrhea, sometimes a sore mouth or mouth ulcers, changes in taste in the mouth and tongue, and changes in smell.
- Chemotherapy can affect the blood stem cells in the bone marrow. The bone marrow stem cells will divide into three different types of blood cells.

  * Red blood cells, which carry oxygen to all parts of the body. If the red blood cell numbers are decreased, then the transportation of oxygen around the body will slow down and the person will develop anemia and feel very tired and lethargic. Sometimes she/he may feel shortness of breath, or feel dizzy and lightheaded because there is less oxygen being carried around the body.

  * White blood cells, which are essential to the immune function for fighting infection and monitoring mutation, among other things. If your white blood cells counts are decreasing, the immune function will decrease and there will be an increased chance of infection.

  * Platelets, which help the blood clot and control bleeding. If your platelet counts are decreasing, you have a high chance of bruising

and you may have a nosebleed or may bleed more than usual from minor cuts or bruises.

- Hair loss: Some chemotherapy can damage the hair and make it brittle or thin, and some chemotherapy can make all of the hair fall out, usually a few weeks into treatment. The body, pubic, and underarm, hair may be lost as well. However, if your hair does fall out due to chemotherapy, it will grow back over a few months once your chemotherapy is finished.
- Skin and nail changes. Skin may become very dry and discolored and more sensitive to sunlight. Nails may grow very slowly or become brittle or flaky.

Long-Term Side Effects

- Chemotherapy's effects on peripheral nerves: Some drugs can cause peripheral polyneuropathy, which is a sensation of tingling, numbness, and pins and needles in your hands or feet. This neuropathy will affect your ability to detect hot or cold objects, which could lead to burns or frostbite, and it can also decrease your sensitivity to the steps you take, which could lead to a fall.
- Chemotherapy's effects on the central nervous system: Long-term use of chemotherapy may cause poor concentration, decreased memory, tinnitus, anxiety, restlessness, dizziness, sleepiness, or headaches.

- Chemotherapy's effects on the kidneys: It can change the kidney function and lead to water retention, loose protein in the urine, or increased BUN and creatinine levels. In order to prevent kidney deterioration, intravenous fluid must be given for several hours before the treatment, and the kidney's functions must be checked before and after each chemotherapy treatment.
- Secondary cancer is another long-term side effect of chemotherapy: Many different types of secondary cancer, such as leukemia, can occur.
- Chemotherapy's effects on fertility: Some chemotherapy treatments may cause infertility. For women, it can sometimes bring on symptoms of menopause and temporarily or permanently stop the ovaries from producing eggs. For men, some chemotherapy drugs may reduce the number of sperm, or affect the sperm's ability to reach and fertilize a woman's egg during intercourse. Some drugs may also, temporarily or permanently, affect the sex life.

TREATMENTS IN TRADITIONAL CHINESE MEDICINE

Traditional Chinese medicine can help with many, but not all, of chemotherapy's side effects. The acupuncture treatments listed below can be helpful with some side effects of chemotherapy.

Gastrointestinal (GI) symptoms

TABLE 34.1

POINTS	MERIDIAN NUMBER	CONDITIONS HELPED
1 Zhong Wan	Ren 12. See Figure 13.3	See Table 13.3
2 Nei Guan	PC 6. See Figure 16.7	See Table 16.1
3 Zu San Li	St 36. See Figure 13.4	See Table 13.3
4 Feng Chi	GB 20. See Figure 12.1	See Table 12.1
5 He Gu	U 4. See Figure 12.3	See Table 12.1
6 Da Zhui	Du 14. See Figure 12.2	See Table 12.1
7 Jin Jing	Extra HN 12. See Figure 26.10	See Table 26.4
8 Yu Ye	Extra HN 13. See Figure 26.10	See Table 26.4
9 Xia Wan	Ren 10. See Figure 34.1	Abdominal pain, diarrhea, indigestion, vomiting
10 Nei Ting	ST 44. See Figure 18.2	See Table 29.1
11 Feng Long	St 40. See Figure 13.3	See Table 13.3
12 Tan Zhong	Ren 17. See Figure 14.2	See Table 14.4
13 Gong Sun	Sp 4. See Figure 21.1	See Table 21.1
14 Ge Shu	UB 17. See Figure 32.5	Vomiting, hiccups, belching, difficulty swallowing, asthma, coughing, spitting up blood, afternoon fever, night sweats, measles
15 Ju Que	Ren 14. See Figure 16.2	See Table 16.1

POINTS	MERIDIAN NUMBER	CONDITIONS HELPED
16 Da Chang Shu	US 25. See Figure 19.1	See Table 19.2
17 San Yin liao	Sp 6. See Figure 16.6	See Table 16.1
18 Shui Dao	St 28. See Figure 26.15	See Table 26.11
19 Gui Lai	St 29. See Figure 26.15	See Table 26.11

Please refer to the accompanying Figures (illustrations) for the locations of the points. And please note that these illustrations are for information only and may not show all the exact locations of the acupuncture points.

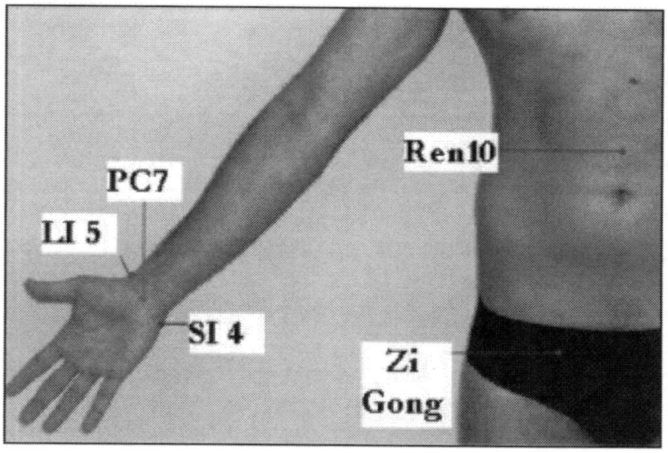

FIGURE 34.1

Gastrointestinal symptoms include nausea, vomiting, gastric regurgitation, tenderness or fullness of the stomach, abdominal pain with very bad breath, also hiccups, diarrhea, and constipation.

- For nausea and vomiting, Zhong Wan, Zu San Li, Nei Guan, He Gu, and Feng Chi are used.
- If a person feels hot and thirsty, it is good to add Da Zhui, Jin Jing, and Yu Ye.

- If the person has bad breath, Xia Wan and Nei Ting are added.
- If there is vomiting of clean water and the person experiences dizziness, Feng Long, Tan Zhong, and Gong Sun are added.
- For hiccups, Ge Shu, and Ju Que are used. If they are accompanied by diarrhea, Ta Chang Shu, Shen Shu, and San Ying Jiao are added.
- For constipation, Feng Long, left Shui Diao, and the left Gui Lai are used.

Fatigue

Chemotherapy can lead the person to feel fatigue, and have shortness of breath, weakness, difficulty walking or standing, heart palpitations, or insomnia.

- The acupuncture points will be Pi Shu, Wei Shu, Zhong Wan, and Zu San Li.
- For heart palpitations and insomnia (poor sleep), Xin Shu, Sheng Men, Ju Que, and San Yin Jiao are added.
- If the person feels cold, has weakness of the lower back and legs, Bui Hui, Da Zhui, Sheng Shu, and Guan Yuan are added.
- If the person feels hot or annoyed, has trouble sleeping, then Fei Shu, Tai Xi, San Yin Jiao are added.

TABLE 34.2

POINTS	MERIDIAN NUMBER	CONDITIONS HELPED
1 Pi Shu	UB 20. See Figure 15.4	See Table 15.2

POINTS	MERIDIAN NUMBER	CONDITIONS HELPED
2 Wei Shu	UB 21. See Figure 31.1	See Table 31.1
3 Zhong Wan	Ren 12. See Figure 13.3	See Table 13.3
4 Zu San Li	St 36. See Figure 13.4	See Table 13.4
5 Xin Shu	UB 15. See Figure 16.3	See Table 16.1
6 Sheng Men	Heart 7. See Figure 29.10	See Table 29.1
7 Ju Que	Ren 14. See Figure 16.2	See Table 16.1
8 San Yin Jiao	Sp 6. See Figure 16.6	See Table 16.1
9 Bai Hui	Du 20. See Figure 22.3	See Table 22.4
10 Da Zhui	Du 14. See Figure 12.2	See Table 12.1
11 Shen Shu	UB 23. See Figure 14.1	See Table 14.4
12 Guan Yuan	Ren 4. See Figure 30.1	See Table 30.1
13 Fei Shu	UB 13 See Figure 13.1	See Table 13.1
14 Tai Xi	Kid 3. See Figure 16.7	See Table 16.2

Please refer to the accompanying Figures (illustrations) for the locations of the points. And please note that these illustrations are for information only and may not show all the exact locations of the acupuncture points.

Menopause and Loss of Fertility

Many people undergoing chemotherapy have impotence, decreased menstruation or menopause, and low libido, accompanied by dizziness, tinnitus, weakness in the low back and knees, and they always feel cold and have insomnia. The treatment is Sheng Shu, Guan Yuan, Qi Men, Zhi Gong, San Yin Jiao, and Zu San Li.

TABLE 34.3

POINTS	MERIDIAN NUMBER	CONDITIONS HELPED
1 Shen Shu	UB 23. See Figure 14.1	See Table 14.4
2 Guan Yuan	Ren 4. See Figure 30.1	See Table 30.1
3 Qi Men	Liver 14 19.2	See Table 19.3
4 Zi Gong	Extraordinary Point. See Figure 34.1	Prolapse of the uterus, irregular menstruation
5 San Yin Jiao	Sp 6. See Figure 16.6	See Table 16.1
6 Zu San Li	St 36. See Figure 13.4	See Table 13.3

Please refer to the accompanying Figures (illustrations) for the locations of the points. And please note that these illustrations are for information only and may not show all the exact locations of the acupuncture points.

Hair Loss

After chemotherapy, many people will have hair loss. Acupuncture can be used to help with this, mainly body acupuncture.

- Tai Xi and Xue Hai, Sheng Men, Feng Chi, Qu Qi, and He Gu.
- Plum Blossom needle, a cluster of 7–9 needles grouped together with a long handle, can be can be used for the hair loss, gently tapping on the scalp until the skin shows slightly redness or mild bleeding. The plum blossom should be used on alternative days, tapping on the scalp for about

twenty minutes. After three or four weeks of treatment, the hair will start to grow gradually, especially in those areas that have lost a patch of hair.

TABLE 34.4

POINTS	MERIDIAN NUMBER	CONDITIONS HELPED
I Tai Xi	Kid 3. See Figure 16.7	See Table 16.2
2 Xue Hai	Sp 10. See Figure 30.1	See Table 30.1
3 Shen Men	Heart 7. See Figure 29.2	See Table 29.1
4 Feng Chi	GB 20. See Figure 12.1	See Table 12.1
5 Qu Qi	LI 11. See Figure 12.2	See Table 12.2
6 He Cu	LI 4. See Figure 12.3	See Table 13.1

Please refer to the accompanying Figures (illustrations) for the locations of the points. And please note that these illustrations are for information only and may not show all the exact locations of the acupuncture points.

Effects on the Central Nervous System (CNS)

After chemotherapy, some people may feel such CNS symptoms as poor concentration, loss of memory, tinnitus, insomnia, nightmares, headaches, or fatigue.

- Acupuncture points for these symptoms will be Zu San Li, Nei Guan, He Gu, Sheng Men, San Ying Jiao, Feng Chi, as well as Bai Hui, Tang Yang, and Tou Wei.

- Another important treatment uses Plum Blossom needles around the cervical, thoracic, and lumbar spine, along the urinary bladder meridians. This is done by tapping from the top and going down three lines following the urinary bladder meridians. Normally, these treatments will greatly improve a person's concentration, memory, and mental function.

TABLE 34.5

POINTS	MERIDIAN NUMBER	CONDITIONS HELPED
1 Zu San Li	St 36. See Figure 13.4	See Table 13.4
2 Nei Guan	PC 6. See Figure 16.7	See Table 16.1
3 He Gu	LI 4. See Figure 12.3	See Table 12.1
4 Shen Men	Heart 7. See Figure 29.2	See Table 29.1
5 San Yin Jiao	Sp 6. See Figure 16.6	See Table 16.1
6 Feng Chi	GB 20. See Figure 12.1	See Table 12.1
7 Bai Hui	Du 20. See Figure 22.3	See Table 22.4
8 Tai Yang	Extra Point. See Figure 22.2	See Table 22.2
9 Tou Wei	St 8. See Figure 22.10	See Table 22.3

Please refer to the accompanying Figures (illustrations) for the locations of the points. And please note that these illustrations are for information only and may not show all the exact locations of the acupuncture points.

Peripheral Polyneuropathy

The long-term side effects of chemotherapy can gradually damage the peripheral nerves. The person may symptomatically feel numbness and a tingling sensation on both the hands and the feet, and may also experience burning, sharp pins and needles along them. The treatments will depend on the location of the condition.

- For the upper extremities, Jian Yu, Jian Liao, Qu Chi, He Gu, Tian Jing, Chi Zhe, and Da Ling, Yang Xi, Wan Gu, Yang Chi, and Wai Guan are used.

TABLE 34.6

POINTS	MERIDIAN NUMBER	CONDITIONS HELPED
1 Jian Yu	LI 15. See Figure 26.6	See Table 26.1
2 Jian Liao	SJ 14. See Figure 34.2	Pain and motor impairment of the shoulder and upper arm
3 Qu Chi	LI 11. See Figure 12.2	See Table 12.2
4 He Gu	LI 4. See Figure 12.3	See Table 12.1
5 Tian Jing	LJ 10. See Figure 34.2	Migraine, pain in the neck, shoulder, and arm, epilepsy
6 Chi Zhe	Lu 5. See Figure 13.2	See Table 13.2
7 Da Ling	PC 7. See Figure 34.1	Cardiac pain, convulsions, epilepsy, foul breath, insomnia, irritability, mental disorders, palpitations, stomach ache, stuffy chest, vomiting
8 Yang Xi	LI 5. See Figure 34.1	Headaches, redness, pain and swelling of the eye, toothache, sore throat, pain of the wrist
9 Wan Gu	SI 4. See Figure 34.1	Headaches, rigidity of the neck, pain in the wrist, jaundice
10 Yang Chi	SJ 4. See Figure 34.2	Pain in the arm, shoulder and wrist, malaria, deafness, thirst

POINTS	MERIDIAN NUMBER	CONDITIONS HELPED
11 Wai Guan	SJ S. See Figure 34.2	See Table 12.2

Please refer to the accompanying Figures (illustrations) for the locations of the points. And please note that these illustrations are for information only and may not show all the exact locations of the acupuncture points.

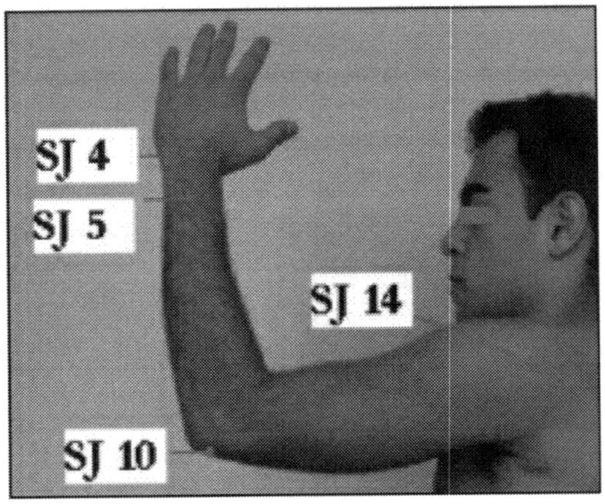

FIGURE 34.2

- For the lower extremities, Huan Tiao, Chi Bian, Cheng Fu, Yang Ling Quan, Du Bi, Liang Qiu, Zu San Li, Kun Lun, Tai Xi, Jie Xi, Qiu Xu, Sheng Mai, and Zao Hai are used.

TABLE 34.7

POINTS	MERIDIAN NUMBER	CONDITIONS HELPED
1 Huan Tiao	GB 30. See Figure 26.8	See Table 26.7
2 Chi Bian	UB 54. See Figure 26.8	See Table 26.2
3 Cheng Fu	UB 36. See Figure 34.3	Bloody stools, diarrhea, dysentery, hemorrhoids, impotence
4 Yang Ling Quan	GB 34. See Figure 15.3	See Table 15.3
5 Du Bi	St 35. See Figure 34.4	Pain, numbness, and motor impairment of the knee

POINTS	MERIDIAN NUMBER	CONDITIONS HELPED
6 Liang Qiu	St 34. See Figure 34.4	Pain and numbness of the knee, gastric pain, motor impairment of the lower extremities
7 Zu San Li	St 36. See Figure 34.4	See Table 13.3
8 Kun Lun	UB 30. See Figure 22.6	See Table 22.1
9 Tai Xi	Kid 3. See Figure 16.7	See Table 16.2
10 Jie Xi	St 41. See Figure 34.4	Pain of the ankle joint, muscular atrophy, motor impairment, pain and paralysis of the lower extremities, epilepsy, headaches, dizziness, and vertigo, abdominal distension, constipation
11 Qiu Xu	GB 40. See Figure 32.2	See Table 32.2
12 Sheng Mai	UB 62. See Figure 29.4	See Table 29.2
13 Zhao Hai	Kid 6. See Figure 34.4	Irregular menstruation, prolapse of uterus, urinary retention, constipation, epilepsy, insomnia, sore throat, asthma

Please refer to the accompanying Figures (illustrations) for the locations of the points. And please note that these illustrations are for information only and may not show all the exact locations of the acupuncture points.

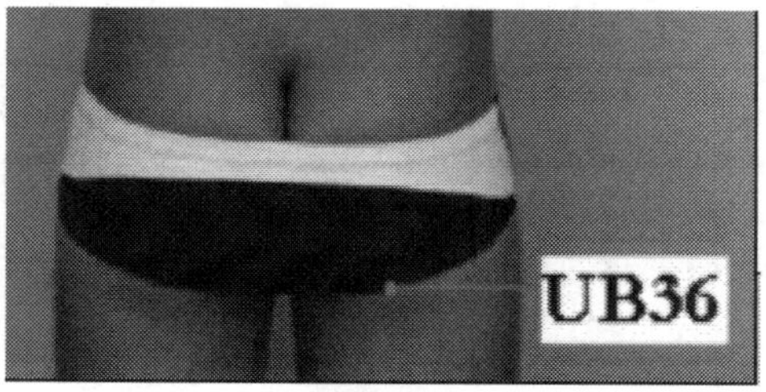

FIGURE 34.3

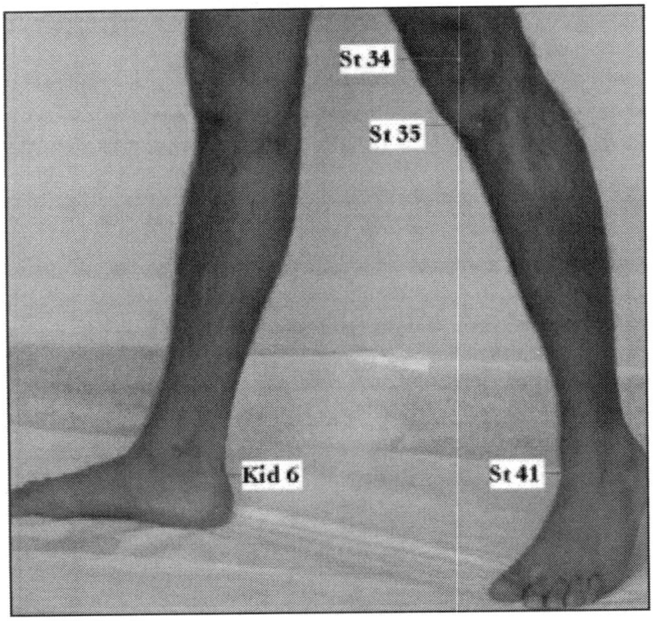

FIGURE 34.4

TREATMENT FOR THE SIDE EFFECTS OF AMANDA'S CHEMOTHERAPY

As you read from the above, Amanda had one of the common side effects of chemotherapy. I first treated her symptoms of pain, depression, and anxiety, with the above-mentioned methods and they are getting better. Then I tried to treat her GI symptoms and fatigue. Although her treatment with me was on, off, and regular, because she was busy going for chemotherapy a few times a week, after my treatments, she feels her appetite is better and her fatigue is much improved. I also treated the numbness and tingling sensation in her hands and toes for about three months, but it proved the most difficult problem to solve as she still felt numbness and tingling after the three months, so she was advised to come to my office once a week to maintain her treatment. The treatments were successful and she finally feels the numbness and tingling has been reduced. Additionally, her energy has been restored enough that she has been able to return to a regular schedule for her work and family life.

TIPS TO USE AT HOME OR OFFICE

- Acupuncture cannot cure cancer. Please be aware of the limitations of acupuncture in this respect.
- However, acupuncture can help a good deal with the side effects of chemotherapy. It is therefore worthwhile to try if you have gastrointestinal symptoms, fatigue, hair loss, infertility, CNS-related problems, or polyneuropathy after chemotherapy.

Glossary

Acupuncture points. (also called **acupoints**) These are locations on the body that acupuncturists focus on when selecting where to insert their needles for the particular illness of the patient. Acupuncture is based on the theories of meridians, which are connected points in the anatomy that affect a specific organ or part of the body, and yin and yang, which is an ancient Chinese philosophy. Other treatment methods, such as acupressure, sonopuncture, and laser acupuncture, also use the acupuncture points to perform their treatment. Around 400 commonly used acupuncture points are located in twelve major meridians. There are also numerous extra points not associated with a particular meridian, but they are very effective for treating many illnesses.

Anihidrosis. The inability to sweat in response to heat.

Channels and Collaterals. The theory of channels and collaterals is an important component of traditional Chinese medicine. It covers physiological functions and pathological changes and is essential in guiding clinical practice, especially acupuncture treatment. Physiologically, they are branches that connect all the meridians into a series of connecting passages through which qi and blood circulate to regulate the functions of the zang-fu organs, tissues, and sense organs. These passages also conduct the sensations and reactions of acupuncture treatment.

DASH (Dietary Approaches to Stop Hypertension) Eating Plan. This plan, known to reduce blood pressure and bad cholesterol, emphasizes fruits, vegetables, and low-fat dairy products, as well as fish, nuts, poultry, and whole grains. It also calls for a reduction in fats, red meat, sweets, and sugar-containing beverages.

Differentiation of syndromes. This is a method of understanding and diagnosing disease by the theories of traditional Chinese medicine (TCM). TCM uses four diagnostic methods: 1) inspection, 2) listening and smelling, 3) inquiring, and [4] palpation, to obtain information from the patients. In combination with the information obtained from the four diagnostic methods, the diagnostic procedure includes an analysis of the clinical data regarding symptoms, physical signs, and disease history.

Etiology. The science that deals with the causes or origin of disease.

Five elements. In traditional Chinese thought, natural phenomena can be classified into five substances or phases—wood, fire, earth, metal, and water. These five phases are not materials, they are metaphors for describing interactions and relationships between phenomena. The doctrine of five phases was employed in many fields of early Chinese thought, including such seemingly disparate fields as music, medicine, martial arts, and military strategy.

Meridians. A series of twelve main and eight secondary pathways that crisscross the body, each named for a particular internal organ. Of the hundreds of strategic points, most are far from the area they are believed to influence.

Moxibustion. A traditional Chinese medicine therapy using moxa, or mugwort herb. Acupuncturists burn the moxa fluff or process it into a stick that resembles a cigar. They can use it indirectly, with acupuncture needles, or sometimes burn it on a patient's skin.

Needling methods. Acupuncturists twist or insert acupuncture needles in a number of ways to induce qi (energy) for the purpose of curing different illnesses.

Pathology. In medicine, pathology is the study and diagnosis of disease. In traditional Chinese medicine, as well, it studies the causes, effects, and nature of diseases.

Qi (pron. *chee*). Vital energy conducted throughout the body by meridians.

Reticular formation. Involved in the waking and sleeping cycle, this chaotic, loose, and intricate form of organization in the brain stem is essential for governing some of the basic functions of higher organisms and appears to be at the crux of basic neurological and behavioral functions of the human being. The cells lack clear ganglionic boundaries, but do have clear functional organizations and distinct cell types. The term *reticular formation* is seldom used any longer except to speak in generalities. Modern anatomy, or neuroscience articles, usually refer to the individual nuclei that comprise the reticular formation.

Traditional Chinese Medicine (TCM). The name given to all aspects of China's medical heritage. It encompasses the medical theory and practices of Chinese medicine, especially herbal medicine, acupuncture, and other methods that prevent or treat illness and promote health and well-being.

Yin-yang theory. A conceptual philosophy of two opposing life forces that was used for observing and analyzing the material world in ancient China.

Zang-fu. A general term for the organs of the human body. It includes six zang organs—the heart, lung, spleen, liver, kidney, and pericardium—and six fu organs—the gallbladder, stomach, small intestine, large intestine, urinary bladder, and San Jiao.

APPENDIX

Tips for Acupuncture Practitioners

Chapter 12—The Common Cold

Wind Cold

- Electrical stimulation at Du 16, GB 20, LI 4, and Lu 7 for 30 minutes will greatly reduce the symptoms.
- This treatment should continue for two days, one session per day.

Wind Heat

- Electrical stimulation at Du 14, SJ 5, LI 4, and Lu 10 for 30 minutes will greatly reduce the symptoms.
- Continue this treatment for two days, one session a day.

Chapter 13—Bronchitis

- Always electrically stimulate UB 13 Fei Shu. If the patient has wind cold, Lu 7 Lie Que and Du 14 Da Zhui. For wind heat, LI 11 Qu Chi and Du 14 Da Zhui.

- Combining UB 13 Fei Shu with St 36 Zu San Li and St 40 Feng Long may greatly improve your patient's immune function.

Chapter 14—Asthma

Excess Type 1—Wind Cold

- Use electrical stimulation on UB 12, UB 13, and Du 14.
- Use an ultra red heating lamp on UB 12, UB 13, and Du 14 for 20–30 minutes.
- UB 13 and UB 12 are located in the vicinity of the lung, which will greatly improve the lung's function and energy and will protect the lung from the attacking pathogens. They will clear the lung and eliminate the wind. DU 14, Lu 7, and L I4 function to eliminate the wind cold and clear the lung, therefore soothing the asthma.

Excess Type 1—Phlegm Heat

- Because phlegm heat shows signs of mild infection of the lung, there are more points to choose from for eliminating the pathogens, such as wind heat.
- Prescription: UB 13 Fei Shu, EX B1 Ding Chuan, Ren 22 Tian Tu, Lu 5 Qi Ze, St 40 Feng Long.

Deficiency Type 2—Lung

- No heating lamp.

- Use these 5 points: UB 13 Fei Shu, Lu 9 Tai Yuan, St 36 Zu San Li, Ren 22 Tian Tu and Sp 3 Tai Bai. and do electrical stimulation for 20–30 minutes. If they are pairs, you should use the paired points also.
- Lu 5 Chi Ze is very important to reduce the phlegm heat and soothe the arm's smooth muscle. Fen Long St 40 is a point of strengthening the spleen function which resolves the problem of phlegm.
- UB 13 Fei Shu is applied to clear the lung and regulate the flow of energy. Ren 22 Tian Tu causes the energy to subside and resolves the problem of phlegm, as well as eliminating excessive heat. Ding Chaun is the point which causes a cessation of wheezing and makes breathing much easier.
- Prescription: UB 13 Fei Shu, Lu 9 Tai Yuan, St 36 Zu San Li, and Sp 3 Tai Bai.

Deficiency Type 2—Kidney

- A heating lamp should be used for UB 23 and UB 13.
- Electrical stimulation for UB 23, Ren 17, and Ren 6.
- Ki 3 Tai Xi strengthens the primary energy of the kidney and, when combined with UB 23 Shen Shu, the original point adjacent to the kidney, it will greatly enhance the Ki 3 functions. Ren 17 Tan Zhong is one of the most important energy

points in the eight influential points and UB 13 Fei Shu is the back-shu point of the lung, which reinforces energy and smooths out ragged breathing. Ren 6 Qi Hai is an important point to reinforce lung energy, recreate energy in the lower lung respiratory track, and also strengthen the kidney and primary energy.

Chapter 15—Allergy and Sinusitis

Type 1 Allergy and Sinusitis

- By electrically stimulating the points of LI 20 Ying Xiang, UB 2 Zan Zhu, and GB 14 Yang Bai, your patients may be pleased and surprised that their sinusitis and headaches go away within one to two sessions. This is because the above points may increase the opening of the sinus and drain it. The patients will feel that the pressure over the sinus is reduced after the treatment.
- LI 20 Ying Xiang is the outlet of the large intestine meridian and is adjacent to the nose, thus LI 20 connects the nose to the sinus after stimulation of the point. Stimulation of points of LI 20, UB 2, and GB 14 desensitizes the mucus membrane and decreases the amount of secretion. Hu Gu is the original location of the large intestine point. It can decrease the invasion of the allergen and can also expel the allergen from the body. GB 20 Feng Chi will enhance LI 4 He Gu in its function to expel the invasion of the allergen.

Type 2 Allergy and Sinusitis

- For allergic eye symptoms, use GB 20 Feng Chi, LI 11 Qu Qi, LI 4 He Gu, plus the following: St 1 Cheng Qi, St 2 Si Bai, SJ 23 Si Zu Kong, GB 14 Yang Bai, GB 1 Tong Zi Liao, UB 2 Zan Zhu, UB 1 Qing Ming, ST 8 Tou Wei, and Ex HN5 Tai Yang.
- For itching in the ear, add SJ 21 Er Meng, SI 19 Ting Gong, and GB 2 Ting Hui.
- Electrical stimulations for SI 19, SJ 21, and GB 2 will greatly improve hearing, tinnitus, and decrease the ear itching. You have to further differentiate the symptoms based on body types. There are two subtypes:
- For kidney yang deficiency, accompanied with symptoms of cold in all 4 extremities, and fatigue, add UB 23 Sheng Shu.
- For gallbladder fire excess, bitterness in the mouth, and inflamed eye, add GB 34 Yang Ling Quan and Li 3 Tai Chong.
- GB 20 Feng Chi protects the patient from the allergen invasion and strengthens the immune function of the body. St 8 Tou Wei and Ex HN5 Tai Yang are placed around the scalp and will decrease headaches.

Chapter 16—Smoking

- Education, education! This is the most important part. If a patient is not willing to quit, there is no way to force that patient to quit.

- Encouragement. You have to encourage the patient to do so.
- Support. You have to get support from the patient's family and friends.

Chapter 18—Gastritis

- Use a heating lamp.
  Place a heating pad on the patient's abdomen.

Chapter 19—Irritable Bowel Syndrome (IBS)

- Place a heating lamp on the stomach for 25 minutes.
- Use electrical stimulation for 25 minutes on Li 14, St 36, St 25, and Rn 6. You may get some unexpected results.

Chapter 21—Weight Control

- The most important issue is to encourage your patient to stick to the program for at least 3–6 months.
- Auricular needles might be useful on their own, without combining with body acupuncture to suppress the appetite.
- A diet program alone might be enough for some patients to lose weight.
- Prevention is always more important than the treatment.

Chapter 22—Headaches

- The most important thing is to identify what meridian headache category your patient belongs to: Tai Yang, Yang Ming, Shao Yang, or Jue Ying.
- Identify the external type, wind cold or wind heat. If you combine the meridian with the external type, your acupuncture effects will be much more successful than the average acupuncturist's.
- The distal points on the hands and feet are very important for your treatment. Please do not ignore these distal points.
- Please put your patients in a quiet room with low illumination, and use electrical stimulation for 30 minutes.
- Many headaches may be triggered by occipital neuralgia, trigeminal neuralgia, the common cold, sinusitis, or allergies. For headaches that are secondary to the above, it is necessary to treat the original trigger—the sinusitis, occipital neuralgia, trigeminal neuralgia, common cold, and allergies. By effectively treating the original trigger of the primary headache, your patient's recovery rate will be much higher than the average acupuncturist's is. For many years, 99 percent of my patients with headache problems have felt much improved after my treatments because I always treat the trigger factors, and not just the headache that results from them.

Chapter 23—Insomnia

- Always use liver points for stress reduction.
- My personal experience: always add EX-HN 1 Si Sheng Cong and Du 20 Bai Hui points for stress reduction, which will greatly improve the sleep quality. I have a patient who slept for 14 hours after his first treatment from me.

Chapter 24—Tinnitus

- Electrical stimulation of SJ 21, SI 19, GB 2, and SJ 17 for 10 minutes per session, 3 times a week for 4–6 weeks will bring good results.
- Liv 3 and Kid 3 are good points for stress reduction in tinnitus.

Chapter 25—Hearing Loss

- In my experience, treatment for hearing loss should be combined with symptoms of other internal organs. For example, if a patient experiences kidney deficiency, it is necessary to treat some of the kidney meridians to enhance the function of the kidney. If the liver or gallbladder show signs of excessive heat, such as a headache, anxiety, or loss of temper, it is necessary to treat some of the points on the liver meridian to decrease the heat. If the patient complains of poor digestion or appetite, it is necessary to treat the spleen and stomach points, which help improve the digestive function, and all these together will help the hearing loss and help the patient recover hearing function.

Chapter 26—Strokes

- Always use acupuncture treatments for both body and scalp.
- Treat your patients with the highest electrical stimulation your patients can tolerate.
- Encourage your patients to avoid the use of any unaffected extremity and instead force them to use the paralyzed body part.
- Based on new studies, patients still have a good chance to recover, even six months after a stroke. Never give up!

Chapter 27—Bell's Palsy

- Put the needles primarily on the paralyzed side, but also put a few needles on the healthy side. This will help the energy flow go through the paralyzed side.
- After acupuncture treatment, a massage for about 10–15 minutes will greatly help the patient's recovery.
- Using these methods, most of the time your patients will have a 90–100-percent recovery. Again, the earlier the treatment, the better the results.

Chapter 29—Bipolar Disorder

- Using Du 26 and Du 23 with strong stimulation will greatly improve your patients' symptoms.
- Du 20 is also a good point for any dian and kuang patients.

Chapter 30—Unexplained Infertility

- According to studies from Germany and Australia, the IVF treatment without acupuncture has a 29-percent success rate for pregnancy. However, the combination of acupuncture with IVF increases the success rate to 49 percent, almost a third higher than IVF alone. Therefore, it would be advisable to combine the two treatments.
- Please tell your patients that persistent treatment is the key, and they should not skip treatment.

Chapter 31—Osteroporosis

- For women above age fifty and men above age sixty, use acupuncture points listed in the chapter once a week. This will greatly improve the calcium and vitamin-D intake from the GI tract.
- Always teach the patient how to prevent falling.
- Encourage the patient to take vitamin D, 1000 IU, and calcium, 1000mg, per day.

Chapter 32—Diabetes

- Controlling the pain is the most important methodology to help diabetic neuropathy. The patient should be treated with increased stimulation by the acupuncture stimulation machine. The level should be set as high as possible and for as long as the patient can tolerate it.
- Large diameter needles should be used for the treatment of nerve pain; the needles should first be put in a shallow position and then gradually put in the full depth. The electrical stimulation machine must be attached to the needles for about thirty minutes.
- You should not only treat the patient's pain, but also other accompanying symptoms, such as sexual, urinary, or GI problems, or dizziness.

Chapter 33—Hypertension

- Keep the patient in a quiet environment for treatment.
- The points on the head are very important. If you have a chance to do so, you can create a mild bleeding from the points on Tai Yang and Yin Tang, and the blood pressure will go down immediately.

Chapter 34—Chemotherapy Symptoms

- The earlier the treatment, the better the results.

- Plum Blossom treatments are very important for hair loss and peripheral polyneuropathy—nerve pain in the extremities.

References

Chapter 1

[1] Editors from Beijing College of Traditional Medicine, Shanghai College of Traditional Medicine, Nanjing College of Traditional Medicine, and the Acupuncture Institute of the Academy of Traditional Chinese Medicine. *Essentials of Chinese Medicine.* Beijing, China: Foreign Language Press, 1980, pp.5ff.

[2] Stevens, Mark A., editor, *Merriam-Webster's Collegiate Encyclopedia.* Springfield, MA: Merriam-Webster, Inc., 2000, p.1723.

Chapter 2

[1] Johnson, MJ. "How Acupuncture Works." *Traditional Chinese Medicine World.* 4(4):1, 2, 3, Winter 2002.

[2] Modica, P. "Physicians Take Acupuncture Mainstream." *Medical Tribune.* 39(16):20, September 17, 1998.

[3] Lee, MHM, Liao, JJ. "Acupuncture: Which Patients Might It Help? An Ancient Chinese Technique Is Finding Its Place In Western Medicine." *Emergency Medicine.* April 1998, pp 18–46.

[4] Sabatino, F. "Mind and Body Medicine: A New Paradigm?" *Hospitals.* February 20, 1993, pp 66–71.

[5] Hong, G G. "Acupuncture: The Historical Basis and Its U.S. Practitioners," *Laboratory Medicine.* 29(3): March 1998, pp 163–166.

[6] Scheck, A. "Acupuncture: More FPs Getting The Point." *Family Practice News.* 22(12):1, 17, June 15, 1992. (Was 9 on orig.)

Chapter 3

[1] Acupuncture. N.I.H. Consensus Statement Online, http://consensus.nih.gov/1997/1997 acupuncture107html 15(5):1–34, Nov 3–5, 1997.

[2] Acupuncture: an introduction. National Center for Complementary and Alternative Medicine, NCCAM Publication, No. D404, http://nccam.nih.gov/health/acupuncture/introduction.htm created December 2007.

[3] Melzack R, Wall, PD. "Pain mechanisms: A new theory." *Science.* 150:171–179, 1965.

[4] Wall, P.D, Melzack, R. "On the nature of cutaneous sensory mechanisms." *Brain,* 85:331–356, 1962.

[5] Melzack, R. "Acupuncture and pain mechanisms." *Anaesthesist.* 25:204–207, 1976.

[6] Ahsin, S, Saleem, S, Bhatti, AM, et al. "Clinical and endocrinological changes after electro-acupuncture treatment in patients with osteoarthritis of the knee." *Pain.* Sept 17, 2009.

[7] Cheng, CH, Yi, PL, Lin, JG, et al. "Endogenous Opiates in the Nucleus Tractus" *Journal of*

Complementary Alternative Medicine. Sep 3, 2009.

[8] Lee, HJ, Lee, JH, Lee, EO et al. "Substance P and beta-endorphin mediate electro-acupuncture induced analgesia in mouse cancer pain model." *Journal of Experimental & Clinical Cancer Research.* 28:102, Jul 16, 2009.

[9] Silberstein, M. "The cutaneous intrinsic visceral afferent nervous system: A new model for acupuncture analgesia." *Journal of Theoretical Biology.* Sept 15, 2009.

[10] Zhang, J, Zhang, N. "Study on mechanisms of acupuncture analgesia." *Z-hongguo Zhen Jiu.* 27(1):72–75, Jan 2, 2007.

[11] Chae, Y, Lee, H, Kim, H, et al. "The neural substrates of verum acupuncture compared to non-penetrating placebo needle: an fMRI study." *Neuroscience Letters.* 450(2):80–84, Jan 30, 2009.

[12] Li, K, Shan B, Xu, J, et al. "Changes in fMRI in the human brain related to different durations of manual acupuncture needling" *Journal of Alternative and Complementary Medicine.* 12(7):615–623, Sept 13, 2006.

[13] Pariente, J, White, P, Frackowiak, RS, et al. "Expectancy and belief modulate the neuronal substrates of pain treated by acupuncture" *Neuroimage.* 25 (4):1161–1167, May 1, 2005.

Chapter 5

[1] "Medical Acupuncture: FAQ. American Academy of Medical Acupuncture" www.medicalacupuncture.org/acu_info/faqs.html accessed October 2009.

[2] Acupuncture. N.I.H. Consensus Statement Online, http://consensus.nih.gov/1997/1997acupuncture107html 15(5):1–34, Nov 3–5, 1997.

Chapter 6

[1] Yang, CP, Hsieh, CL, Wang, NH, et al. "Acupuncture in patients with carpal tunnel syndrome: A randomized controlled trial" *Clinical Journal of Pain.* 25(4):327–333, May 2009.

[2] Witt, CM, Jena, S, Brinkhaus, B, et al. "Acupuncture in patients with osteoarthritis of the knee or hip: a randomized, controlled trial with an additional non-randomized arm". *Arthritis & Rheumatism.* 54(11):3485–3493, Nov 2006.

[3] Berman, BM, Lao, L, Langenberg, P, et al. "Effectiveness of acupuncture as adjunctive therapy in osteoarthritis of the knee: a randomized, controlled trial." *Annals of Internal Medicine.* 141(12):901–910, Dec 21, 2004.

[4] Yaman, LS, Kiliç, S, Sarica, K, et al. "The place of acupuncture in the management of psychogenic impotence." *European Urology.* 26(1):52–55, 1994.

[5] Engelhardt, PF, Daha, LK, Zils, T, et al. "Acupuncture in the treatment of psychogenic erectile dysfunction: first results of a prospective randomized placebo-controlled study." *International Journal of Impotency Research.* 15 (5):343–346, Oct 2003.

[6] Dieterle, S, Li, C, Greb, R, et al. "Prospective randomized placebo-controlled study of the effect of acupuncture in infertile patients with severe oligoasthenozoospermia." *Fertility and Sterility.* 92(4):1340–1343, Oct 2009.

[7] Manheimer, E, Zhang, G, Udoff, L, et al. "Effects of acupuncture on rates of pregnancy and live birth among women undergoing in vitro fertilisation: systematic review and meta-analysis. *British Medical Journal.* 336(7643):545–549, Mar 8, 2008.

[8] Magarelli, PC, Cridennda, DK, Cohen, M. "Changes in serum cortisol and prolactin associated with acupuncture during controlled ovarian hyperstimulation in women undergoing in vitro fertilization-embryo transfer treatment." *Fertility and Sterility.* Dec 30, 2008.

[9] Dieterle, S, Ying, G, Hatzmann, W, et al. "Effect of acupuncture on the outcome of in vitro fertilization and intracytoplasmic sperm injection: a randomized, prospective, controlled clinical study." *Fertility and Sterility.* 85 (5):1347–1351, May 2006.

[10] Siterman, S, Eltes, F, Schechter, L, et al. "Success of acupuncture treatment in patients with initially low sperm output is associated with a decrease in scrotal skin temperature." *Asian Journal of Andrology.* 11(2):200–208, Mar 2009.

[11] Cherkin, DC, Sherman, KJ, Avins, AL, et al. "A randomized trial comparing acupuncture, simulated acupuncture, and usual care for chronic low back pain. *Archives of Internal Medicine.* 169(9):858–866, May 11, 2009.

[12] Ezzo, JM, Richardson, MA, Vickers, A, et al. "Acupuncture-point stimulation for chemotherapy-induced nausea or vomiting" *Cochrane Database System Review.* (2):CD002285, Apr 19, 2006.

[13] Lee, A, Done, ML. "Stimulation of the wrist acupuncture point P6 for preventing postoperative nausea and vomiting" *Cochrane Database System Review.* 17.CD003281, 2004. Update in: *Cochrane Database System Review.* (2):CD003281, 2009.

[14] Chan, DK, Johnson, MI, Sun, KO, et al. "Electrical acustimulation of the wrist for chronic neck pain: a randomized, sham-controlled trial using a wrist-ankle acustimulation device." *Clinical Journal of Pain.* 25(4):320–326, May 2009.

[15] Trinh, K, Graham, N, Gross, A, et al. "Acupuncture for neck disorders." *Spine.*

(Philadelphia, Pa 1976). 32(2):236–343, Jan 15, 2007.

[16] Irnich, D, Behrens, N, Molzen, H, et al. "Randomised trial of acupuncture compared with conventional massage and 'sham' laser acupuncture for treatment of chronic neck pain." *British Medical Journal.* 323(7324):1306–1307, Dec 1, 2001.

[17] Sato, M, Inubushi, M, Shiga, T, et al. "Therapeutic effects of acupuncture in patients with rheumatoid arthritis: a prospective study using (18)F-FDG-PET." *Annals of Nuclear Medicine.* 23(3):311–316, May 2009.

[18] Liu, XD, Zhang, JL, Zheng, HG, et al. "Clinical randomized study of bee-sting therapy for rheumatoid arthritis" [Article in Chinese.] *Zhen Ci Yan Jiu.* 33(3):197–200, June 2008.

[19] Lathia, AT, Jung, SM, Chen, LX. "Efficacy of acupuncture as a treatment for chronic shoulder pain" *Journal of Alternative Complementary Medicine.* 15(6):613–618, June 2009.

[20] Bier, ID, Wilson, J, Studt, P, et al. "Auricular acupuncture, education, and smoking cessation: a randomized, sham-controlled trial" *American Journal of Public Health.* 92(10):1642–1647, October 2002.

[21] Yan, T, Hui-Chan, CW. "Transcutaneous electrical stimulation on acupuncture points improves muscle function in subjects after acute stroke: a randomized controlled trial." *Journal*

of Rehabilitative Medicine. 41 (5):312–316, April 2009.

[22] Trinh, KV, Phillips, SD, Ho, E, et al. "Acupuncture for the alleviation of lateral epicondyle pain: a systematic review" *Rheumatology* (Oxford), 43(9):1085–1090, September 2004.

Chapter 7

[1] "Acupuncture: Can It Help?" Mayo Clinic Health Information. Rochester, MN, 2007.

[2] Kidson, R. *Acupuncture for Everyone.* Rochester, VT: Healing Arts Press, 2000, p 160.

Chapter 34

[1] U.S. Cancer Statistics Working Group. United States Cancer Statistics: 1999–2005 Incidence and Mortality Web-based Report. Atlanta (GA): Department of Health and Human Services, Centers for Disease Control and Prevention, and National Cancer Institute, 2009. Available at: www.cdc.gov/uscs

[2] Note: Incidence counts cover approximately 96 percent of the U.S. population and death counts cover 100 percent of the U.S. population. Use caution in comparing incidence and death counts.

Resources

Chinese Acupuncture and Moxibustion. Editor in Chief, Cheng Xinnong, Beijing Foreign Languages Press, 1987.

Miraculous Skills in Traditional Chinese Acupuncture and Moxibustion. Editor in Chief, Shi Xue-Min, Tianjing Scientific and Translation Press, 1992.

Chinese Acupuncture Prescription Collection. Editor in Chief, Wang Lizhao, Jiangxi Scientific and Technology Press, 1990.

About the Authors

Jun Xu, M.D., L.Ac.

Dr Jun Xu is a medical doctor in Connecticut specializing in rehabilitative medicine and acupuncture in his private practice and as an attending physician in the department of Physical Medicine and Rehabilitation at Stamford Hospital. He spent eight years training in traditional Chinese medicine (TCM) and acupuncture, and received his medical degree and master of medicine from two medical schools in China. He then taught and practiced medicine and acupuncture at Guangzhou College of Chinese Medicine in China.

In the 1980s, Xu migrated to America, and became a Postdoctoral Research Fellow, first at the University of Georgia, then at Albert Einstein College of Medicine in the Bronx, New York. He interned for a year at St. Francis Medical Center in Pittsburgh, Pa, then transferred to the New York Medical College in Valhalla, where he received his three-year resident training in Physical Medicine and Rehabilitation. After graduation, he started his private practice in both physical medicine and acupuncture. He is also an Attending Physician and Acupuncturist at the Heart and Vascular Institute of Stamford Hospital. In that capacity, he worked with a well-known thoracic surgeon, administering acupuncture treatments before and after thoracic surgery, as well as other departments in the hospital.

Dr. Xu is certified by the American Board of Physical Medicine and Rehabilitation. He is a Diplomat in Acupuncture and Chinese Herbology, certified by NCCAOM, the National Commission for the Certification of Acupuncture and Oriental Medicine, and has Acupuncture and M.D. Physician licenses in several states, including Connecticut.

His medical society memberships include the American Academy of Physical Medicine and Rehabilitation and The Association of Chinese American Physicians (ACAP). Since March 2010, he has been president of the American Traditional Chinese Medicine Society (ATCMS) where he had previously served as vice president.

Dr. Xu has been featured in magazines and on several television shows. In addition, he has lectured and has published a significant number of research articles for medical journals. He lives in Scarsdale, New York with his wife and children.

More information can be found at http://drxuacupuncture.com/ or www.rmac.yourmd.com/

Frank Murray

A former editor of *Better Nutrition, GreatLife, and Let's Live (England),* Frank Murray is the author or coauthor of fifty books on health and nutrition, including *100 Super Supplements for a Longer Life* (available in English and Chinese from McGraw-Hill), and *You Must Eat Meat,* with Max Ernest Jutte, M.D., published by Hutton Electronic Publishing, Westport, CT. His books for Basic Health Publications include *Sunshine and Vitamin D, Natural Supplements for Diabetes, Health Benefits Derived from Sweet Orange, Ampalaya: Nature's Remedy for Type 1 and Type 2 Diabetes,* and *How to Prevent Prostate Problems.*

In 2006, he was awarded the National Nutritional Foods Association's President's Award in Las Vegas. A member of the New York Academy of Sciences, Mr. Murray lives in New York.

Made in United States
Orlando, FL
04 November 2026

90202365R00234